Dec 20, 2012

Dusan

Best

Khalil

M000236386

Don't Let Your Heart Attack!

A comprehensive guide to help you understand heart disease, cholesterol metabolism and learn how to take charge of implementing your personal cardiovascular disease prevention, treatment and reversal strategies

by

K. H. Sheikh, MD, MBA

Fellow of the American College of Cardiology
Diplomate of the American Board of Clinical Lipidology

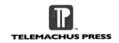

TELEMACHUS PRESS

Cover Designed by Telemachus Press, LLC

Cover art:
Copyright © Thinkstock/90996452/istockphoto
Copyright © Thinkstock/200247896-001/photodisc

Images:
Figure 2.1: Image Copyright © 9134923/Shutterstock.com
Figure 2.2: Image Copyright © 76383646/Shutterstock.com
Figure 2.3: Image Copyright © 91560044/Shutterstock.com
Figure 2.4: Image Copyright © 78383649 /Shutterstock.com
Figure 2.5: Image Copyright © 76739923 /Shutterstock.com
Figure 2.6: Image Copyright Alyssia Sheikh
Figure 3.1: Image Copyright Alyssia Sheikh
Figure 3.2: Image Copyright Alyssia Sheikh
Figure 4.1: Image Copyright © 82143466/Shutterstock.com
Figure 4.2: Image Copyright © 80984965 /Shutterstock.com
Figure 4.3: Image Copyright Alyssia Sheikh
Figure 4.4: Image Copyright Alyssia Sheikh
Figure 4.5: Image Copyright Alyssia Sheikh

Published by Telemachus Press, LLC
http://www.telemachuspress.com

Visit the authors website
http://www.sheikheartcare.com

ISBN: 978-1-938135-85-9 (eBook)
ISBN: 978-1-938135-86-6 (Paperback)
ISBN: 978-1-938135-87-3 (Hardback)

Version 2012.11.09

Printed in the United States of America

10 9 8 7 6 5 4 3 2 1

DEDICATION AND ACKNOWLEDGEMENTS

This book is dedicated to my parents. My mother, Izzat nurtured my calling to medicine. My father, Hasan saw to it that I answered the calling.

This book could not have been written without the support of my family. Through my wife, DJ's encouragement, critique and guidance, I remained committed to researching and writing, even after a particularly grueling day of seeing patients or having been on call the previous night. My two younger daughters, Nadia and Laila are my beacons in the dark, seeing to it that I maintain perspective and balance. My oldest daughter, Alyssia not only inspired me, but generously gave of her time, skills, expertise and artistry in helping me to produce the book.

My thanks go to my immediate and extended family and friends, as well as my colleagues, practice partners, office and hospital staff for their understanding as I took time to research and write at their expense and through their largesse. The editing and production staffs of Telemachus press became not only my business partners, but were simultaneously on the list of my most treasured friends and harshest critics. I thank them for being both.

Individual recognitions and thanks go to Ms. Leslie Becker of Cape Canaveral Hospital, who was an invaluable resource in my research. My lifelong friends, Steve and Mary Podnos deserve special mention. Their cajoling and guidance helped me to keep my eye on the target. My sister, Asifa provided much appreciated counsel and advice.

Finally, the book belongs to my patients. From the beginning, it has always been about them. The covenant of caring for them with integrity, compassion and professionalism has been the driving force in my 30-year career. That experience makes me anxious to get started with the next 30 years.

DISCLAIMERS AND CREDITS

Disclaimer: This book is solely for informational and educational purposes, and is not intended as medical advice. It is not a replacement for qualified and professional medical care. Individuals with diagnosed cardiovascular disease and/or those at risk for cardiovascular disease should always consult with their personal health care provider before undertaking any of the lifestyle, dietary or nutritional changes discussed in this book. Likewise, medications, supplements and vitamins discussed in this book are for general reference and are not intended to replace the individualized guidance from your personal health care provider. Although every effort has been made to provide accurate and up-to-date information, this document cannot be guaranteed to be free of factual error. All of the recommendations set forth in this book are supported by research. Nevertheless, this book ultimately represents the opinion of its author. Each individual should consult with their personal health care provider regarding the applicability of any information in this book to their unique medical issues and condition. The author and publisher make no claim to be rendering medical, health or professional services, and take no responsibility for any consequences that may arise, either directly or indirectly, from following the advice set forth in these pages.

All of the medical information pertaining to Tim Russert cited in this book was obtained from sources in the public domain, and does not represent any protected health information.

Credits: Attributions and copyright are designated for each illustration. All images are obtained under license from Shutterstock.com or are original copyrighted work of Alyssia Sheikh, BFA.

TABLE OF CONTENTS

Don't Let Your Heart Attack!

Introduction

ON FRIDAY, JUNE *13, 2008, 58-year-old Tim Russert was at his NBC News offices in Washington, D.C., preparing for his Sunday news program, "Meet the Press." The hard-nosed and affable Russert had hosted the popular program for the past 16 years. At 1:30 p.m., he suddenly felt ill, cried out his last words— "What's happening?"—and collapsed. He was immediately attended to by colleagues, who performed CPR, and rushed to a nearby hospital, where resuscitative measures were unsuccessful.*

An autopsy revealed that Russert had died of a ruptured cholesterol plaque in the left coronary artery. The ruptured plaque resulted in a blood clot in the artery, which cut off the blood supply to the heart, causing Russert's heart to stop.

Russert had been treated by his physicians for low-grade coronary heart disease. He had a stress test two months earlier that was normal. He was on statin medication for high cholesterol, and had lowered his so-called bad cholesterol, the LDL, to 67 mg/dL, the exact level recommended by all U.S. national health care policy boards. By all conventional criteria, he was considered a low-risk patient, and both he and his doctors had done everything right ...

As tragic as the sudden death of Tim Russert was, it is one of the most common, and the single-most feared, ways in which heart disease becomes evident. Although his untimely death was not predictable, Russert remained at risk for heart disease despite receiving top-notch medical care. As you go through this book, you will come to understand what this risk was, and by

i

the time you reach Chapter 15, where the rest of the Russert story is revealed, you will see why top-notch medical care by itself is often not enough to prevent what happened to Russert.

There are multiple medical conditions, genetic predispositions and environmental influences that increase the risk of heart disease. However, the one risk that underlies the development of nearly all heart and circulatory disorders is created by abnormalities in blood cholesterol. Today we know that this means more than just a high cholesterol level. If you are among the 100 million Americans who have cholesterol disorders, then you either already have, or are at risk for developing, heart and circulatory problems. This book is for you.

Why Should You Choose This Book?

In the United States, public policy guidelines from the National Cholesterol Education Program (NCEP) are periodically updated and incorporated into standards of medical practice. It is typically from these guidelines that your health care provider determines your level of risk for developing heart disease and how to evaluate and treat you to lower that risk. This is what determines the standard of care in cholesterol and heart disease management. In this book, you will learn that while these guidelines are very effective at the public health level, they are not very effective at an individualized level.

There are excellent books on the topic of heart disease and cholesterol available to the public that come from renowned academic institutions. The authors of these books are experts who spend their careers doing research, publishing papers and lecturing about heart disease. These experts follow and study the data from subjects enrolled in clinical trials, the results of which help formulate our approaches to diagnosing and treating heart disease.

This book offers an alternative perspective, that of a practicing cardiologist and expert in cholesterol disorders. Instead of following and studying research subjects, I have spent the last 30 years treating patients. You will hear the same practical knowledge and advice that I have imparted to my patients, which has helped to keep them living well, out of the hospital, out of the emergency room and out of the operating room.

One cannot practice preventative cardiology at a high level without knowing the science and maintaining the expertise and credentials that attest to one's abilities. However, the day-to-day practice of cardiology affords an opportunity to extend the knowledge of scientific principles into practical applications in patients. Furthermore, the additional knowledge that comes from having the opportunity to follow the course of those patients for years is the advantage that this book will give you.

To appreciate what a personalized approach to preventing, treating and reversing heart disease means, you will need to understand the science behind heart disease. Therefore, this book is not simplistic or "dumbed-down" for the reader. On the contrary, this book is scientific, and all of the information presented is evidence-based. This book is not a *Cholesterol for Dummies* or *The Idiots Guide to Heart Disease*. It is meant to be a sophisticated and in-depth guide to provide you with a fundamental understanding of cholesterol and the development of arterial plaque or atherosclerosis, and the measures that you can implement to help you prevent, treat and help reverse your heart disease.

Taking Control of Your Heart Risk

One of the most important lessons I have learned from the last 30 years of practicing medicine is that the patients who are most successful in battling heart disease, no matter the treatment approach, are those who become active participants in their care and do not just passively and blindly follow a doctor's advice. What does it mean to be an active participant in your health? It means taking a direct and vigorous interest in knowing as much as you can about your medical condition, your treatment and your prognosis.

Unfortunately, sometimes patients with this attitude and interest in their health are dismissed by their health care providers as busybodies or "difficult." I think the exact opposite; to show such interest means you care about your health enough to want to understand your condition, as well as what options you have for treatment. It means you want to be involved in the decisions that affect your well-being and that you are willing to take responsibility to optimize your health with the guidance and advice of your doctor. It is exactly these types of patients that most really good doctors welcome and look forward to seeing, because in this situation we have a true partnership for improving that patient's health. As I have often said to patients, "There is something wrong if I care more about your health than you do yourself."

Many people shy away from being active participants in their health care. There are many reasons for this, including: (1) they think they might offend the doctor, (2) they believe "that is what I pay the doctor to do," or (3) they believe "it is too technical and too hard to understand all of the medical lingo." I can respond by saying that if your doctor is offended that you take an active interest in your health, find a new doctor. If you solely delegate all of the responsibility of keeping yourself healthy to your doctor, you will fail.

As far as the technical aspects and medical lingo go, there is no doubt that the practice of medicine in this day and age is very sophisticated and complex. This is especially the case in cardiology and cholesterol metabolism, where the pace of innovation, information and research is especially brisk. However, as I have said to my patients countless times, "If I cannot explain the basic aspects of your problem to you in a way that you can understand, and assist you in making informed decisions in your own health care, then that is my failing ... not yours."

Using this Book to Help You Help Yourself

It is my goal in the upcoming chapters to help you build a foundation of knowledge about heart disease by presenting relatively technical ideas with a simple and common sense approach. I will use illustrations, analogies and references to concepts and situations familiar to all of us to achieve this goal. However, I have not changed the concepts, terms or data to simplify them, because you deserve the credit and consideration for accepting the challenge to address this very important health issue at a very high level.

INTRODUCTION

The sequence of chapters is intended to let you acquire the necessary knowledge in a step-wise approach. Part I consists of chapters that discuss the basic anatomy, biology and chemical concepts about cholesterol and atherosclerosis. This is followed by Part II, which lays a foundation for understanding the clinical aspects in the diagnosis of lipid disorders and atherosclerosis. The final section, Part III, discusses various approaches to treatment and prevention. The final chapter helps you design your personalized heart disease prevention, treatment and reversal program; it includes a checklist of important items in your health plan that you can use for discussion with your doctor.

The knowledge you acquire will be relevant to you, because you have bought this book in order to learn enough about your heart and circulation to help either yourself or your spouse, parents, children or anybody else you care about. When you are done, you won't be able to practice medicine, but you will know enough about the basic concepts involving your own heart health so that you can make informed decisions and be your own advocate. In fact, what other aspect of our lives should be a more important motivator than wanting to achieve and maintain good health?

This book is not for all of the 100 million Americans who are at risk for, or already have, heart disease. It is for the select few of you who truly believe that the investment of time and effort in becoming well informed will pay dividends in helping you keep your heart healthy. If you are ready for the challenge, let's go to work so you **"Don't Let Your Heart Attack!"**

PART I
The ABCs: Anatomy, Biology and Chemistry of Cholesterol and Atherosclerosis

Chapter 1
Lies, Damn Lies and Statistics:
The Facts about Heart Disease

HEART DISEASE CAUSED by atherosclerosis, which is the medical term for the occurrence of plaque in arteries, is preventable. That bears repeating. Today, in the 21st century, you are by and large in control of your own destiny when it comes to the risk of developing heart disease. There are few medical illnesses for which we can make that statement. We don't know how to prevent most types of cancer. We don't know how to prevent most common viral illnesses. We don't know how to prevent osteoporosis. The list goes on and on. That is not to say that we don't know what causes these diseases, or how to detect these diseases early, or even things you can do to reduce your risk of developing these illnesses. But aside from using immunizations to prevent many infectious diseases, there are no common illnesses today for which we can make the claim that they are largely preventable through awareness and taking individual action and responsibility.

So there you have it. You don't have to play the hand you were dealt, but rather you can pick and choose which cards you will have and how to play them. To elaborate, and with emphasis: *cardiovascular disease of the type we most typically see causing heart attacks, strokes, angina, heart failure, blood vessel aneurysms and gangrene due to poor circulation, can be prevented.*

It is well known that the selective use of statistics can support any specific point of view, even if this point of view may be misleading. Unfortunately, the statistics supporting the magnitude of the burden of heart disease afflicting modern society are all too real. In this chapter you will see some of these startling statistics. You will be alarmed over the data that indicates this burden will continue to increase during your lifetime. However, you will also see remarkable information from scientific studies that support the concept that heart disease can be prevented and reversed through fairly simple measures that are in your control.

The 20th-Century Epidemic of Heart Disease

For an illness that is preventable, no matter whether you look at it from an individual, community, national or global perspective, we are doing a miserable job. Heart disease became a global epidemic in the 20th century and will become an increasing concern as we go further into the 21st century. What is most astounding is that atherosclerotic heart disease was virtually unknown until 300 years ago, and has become the leading killer in some underdeveloped countries within just one generation.

What we mean by heart disease caused by atherosclerosis is most appropriately called coronary heart disease, or CHD. The leading cause of death and disability globally, CHD already accounts for over 30 percent of all deaths worldwide, and that percentage is increasing. Fourteen million people died of CHD in 1990, 17 million in 2000, and by 2020 that number will be 25 million.

In the United States, according to the American Heart Association, in 2008 there were 14 million people, or about one in 20 Americans, with confirmed CHD. In the U.S., a heart attack occurs in 1.5 million people every year. More than 500,000 Americans die of a heart attack each year. Over half of heart attacks, or about 700,000, occur in somebody who had no previous knowledge that they even had heart disease.

Alert! In 25 percent of individuals with CHD, their first symptom of heart disease is also their last, because they suffer either a fatal heart attack or the syndrome of sudden cardiac death caused by a sudden and catastrophic heart arrhythmia leading to total body collapse. Thus, in the United States, 300,000 people die each year due to heart disease, never knowing that they had a heart problem and never having had an opportunity to correct it.

In developed Western countries there have been considerable advances in the treatment of CHD. Through these advances we have actually seen a significant drop in the likelihood of a person dying due to CHD. Between the years 1980 and 2001, 250,000 fewer Americans died of CHD, a remarkable 46 percent drop in mortality rate. There are many reasons for the improvement in survival rates from CHD. These include advances in medical technology and research that have proven the value of better and earlier diagnostic techniques and better treatments, including medications, heart stents, surgery and defibrillators. There have also been significant advances in convincing people to adopt a better lifestyle. For instance, in the United States from 1980 to 2001, there was a 30 percent drop in the number of people who smoked, a four percent drop in average blood pressure, a six percent drop in average cholesterol levels and an eight percent increase in physical activity.

However, these improvements have been offset by an increase in the incidence of smoking in young people, obesity and diabetes. Even though 30 percent fewer people are smoking, among teenagers and young adults the incidence of cigarette use is increasing dramatically. The incidence of obesity in children and adolescents has increased by 300 percent since 1980. In 2010, 25 percent of all children in the United States were classified as overweight and 11 percent as obese. There were an estimated 25 million diabetics in the United States, or about eight percent of the population. Particularly alarming is the trend showing that an additional two million Americans are developing diabetes every year.

Alert! It is projected that by the year 2050, 15 percent of the U.S. population, or twice the current percentage, will be diabetic. There is a one in three chance that a child born in 2000 will develop diabetes during his or her lifetime.

As a result, even though we can now save more people from dying due to CHD, there are more people now than ever before who are developing CHD. More people are having nonfatal CHD events, such as heart attacks, that they survive. These patients often go on to develop chronic CHD ill-nesses like congestive heart failure and angina. By the age of 60, one in five men and one in 17 women will have CHD. And that is just the tip of the iceberg. It is estimated that simply because of an increase in rates of obesity in the United States, the prevalence of CHD will increase by 5–16 percent by 2035. The aging of the "baby boomer" generation is also expected to have a dramatic effect on the incidence of CHD. People age 75 years and above are already the fastest growing segment of the population. Of people over the age of 75, 40 percent already have CHD, and it is estimated that this segment of the population will contribute to an additional 50 percent of cases of CHD by 2030.

Heart Disease Is Preventable

If we look at what is happening in developing countries of the world, we can learn much about how CHD develops, and also gain some insight into what we can do to prevent it. In 1960 the incidence of CHD in India was one percent. In 1995 it was up to ten percent. In contrast to the dropping mortality rates in the United States mentioned earlier, in Russia the CHD mortality rates for men between the ages of 55 and 60 increased by 55 per-cent between the years 1984 and 2002. In Beijing, China, the CHD mortality rate for men increased by 50 percent and for women increased by 27 percent between the years 1984 and 1999.

What's going on in India, Russia and China? One contributing factor is that these societies, only within the last generation, have gained access to inexpensive, energy-dense, high-calorie, low-fiber diets. These diets contain highly processed foods, often in the form of fast food and snacks. This change in diet has greatly contributed to a rising incidence of obesity, diabetes and cholesterol disorders. For instance, in the Chinese population the average total cholesterol reading rose by 24 percent between the years 1983 and 1993.

A sedentary lifestyle is the other major contributor to CHD. This is highlighted by another Chinese study that showed that in 1989, 84 percent of Chinese households did not own a vehicle. By 1997 this number was down to 70 percent. In those Chinese households with vehicles, the men of the household were twice as likely to develop obesity as were the men in households without vehicles.

Thus, combining western diets with western conveniences and lifestyles has played a major role in the rising incidence and harmful effects of CHD in the developing world. The other point, of course, is that by understanding this phenomenon, we clearly have the ability to take action to control and alter our risk of developing CHD.

In fact, the scientific evidence for this has been around for a long time. One of the earliest scientific studies to investigate the effect of diet and rates of CHD was the Seven Countries Study, published in 1958. The study followed 12,000 middle-aged men and found that diets high in saturated fats, such as those in the United States and Finland, seemed to correspond to a populace having high blood cholesterol and a high prevalence of CHD. In contrast, diets low in saturated fat, such as those in Greece and Japan, were associated with lower blood cholesterol and a lower prevalence of CHD.

Multiple studies have now confirmed and extended the observations that dietary changes alone can profoundly influence prognosis in patients with CHD. In 1989, a diet study from Wales, called the Diet and Reinfarction Trial (DART), demonstrated that in 2,000-plus men who

survived a heart attack, the group of men who ate a diet low in saturated fat
and rich in the polyunsaturated omega-3 fats, had a 29 percent less chance
of dying than men who were told to just restrict saturated fats. Similar
findings came out of the 1999 French Lyon Heart Study that examined 605
men and women who had survived a heart attack. In this study, subjects
were counseled to follow a diet low in saturated fats. They were then compared to the experimental group who followed a diet rich in fruits, vegetables, grains, legumes, olive oil, fish and red wine. The latter group showed a
73 percent reduction in death due to CHD compared to the former. More
recently, in 2003, these findings were confirmed by the GISSI-P Trial
(Gruppo Italiano per lo Studio della Sopavivienza nell'Infarto
Miocardisco—Prevenzione) conducted on 11,000-plus subjects in Italy. The
group that followed a Mediterranean-type diet had a 51 percent reduction in
CHD mortality.

While these diet studies established that it is possible to lower the risk
of dying from CHD in individuals who already have CHD, what is the risk
of developing CHD in people never previously afflicted? This question was
asked and conclusively answered in the MRFIT trial. This study followed
more than 300,000 men with no previous CHD over six years. Initially
published in 1986, this study showed that those individuals with the most
favorable levels of cholesterol and blood pressure, and who did not smoke,
have diabetes or previous CHD, had a 75 percent lower risk of developing
CHD events, such as heart attack, stroke, angina, heart failure, bypass surgery or death, than patients who had unfavorable CHD risk factors.
Recently an analysis of the same study updated after 25 years of follow-up
has confirmed that those same men with the fewest CHD risk factors have
nearly a 90 percent lower risk of dying.

The INTERHEART study from 2004 provides powerful scientific
data to support the premise that only a few CHD risk factors contribute to
the risk of developing CHD. In this study, 28,000 individuals with and
without heart disease were followed from 52 countries over a four-year
period. The principal findings of this study were that nine risk factors
accounted for 90 percent of the cases of study participants going on to have
a heart attack. Those factors are: (1) abnormal blood lipids, (2) smoking, (3)
hypertension, (4) diabetes, (5) abdominal obesity, (6) psychosocial stress, (7)

inadequate consumption of fruits and vegetables, (8) consumption of either too low or excessive quantities of alcohol, and (9) lack of regular physical activity. Of these nine risk factors, smoking and abnormal blood lipids accounted for 70 percent of the heart attacks. The most powerful single factor, that accounted for 50 percent of the heart attack cases, was an abnormal blood lipid pattern, specifically one in which the good cholesterol/bad cholesterol ratio was abnormal.

CHD and the same atherosclerosis process that occurs in other blood vessels outside the heart, including the brain, aorta and blood vessels to the legs and vital organs, is largely a disease of lifestyle and behavior. The Nurses' Health Study, published in 2000 in the prestigious *New England Journal of Medicine*, looked at the question of whether women without a history of any previous heart problems can reduce their future risk of CHD by simply lifestyle modifications. The results of this study showed a remarkable 85 percent reduction in CHD risk over 14 years of follow-up in women who maintained an appropriate weight, ate a healthy diet, had regular physical activity, did not smoke and consumed moderate amounts of alcohol.

The benefits of physical activity are well recognized in reducing CHD events in both men and women. Exercise helps an individual to maintain a healthy weight, blood pressure and blood lipids and reduces the chance of developing diabetes. Exercise also reduces inflammation in the blood vessels and helps to keep the lining of the blood vessels healthier, two important aspects of CHD that will be covered in later chapters. In fact, the benefits of a healthy lifestyle are present whether or not patients take prescribed blood pressure or lipid medications.

The Medical Community and the Health care System Share the Blame

The scientific evidence states very loudly and clearly that it is possible to prevent CHD in most patients who don't already have CHD, and that it is possible to both prevent progression and cause reversal of CHD in patients who already have CHD. This evidence is as robust and solid as any concept in medicine today. Why is it then that we have so many people with CHD, so many new heart attacks and strokes, and why does CHD continue to be the largest cause of mortality in the world?

There are of course a number of reasons. These include: (1) the cost of and access to treatment, (2) adherence to diet, exercise and medication regimens, (3) emergence of new at-risk populations due to the increase in diabetes and childhood obesity, an aging population and an increase in cigarette use among younger adults, (4) inadequate attention to or inadequate recognition of additional CHD risk factors, (5) concerns about medication safety, and (6) lack of counseling and implementation of well-established treatment guidelines by health care practitioners. Some of these obstacles are at public health and societal levels. However, many are in the control of the individual, that being YOU.

The importance of making it your own responsibility to know your CHD risk and know what to do to prevent and reverse CHD has never been more important than now. Multiple studies now confirm the poor job that our health care system does in lifestyle counseling and emphasizing preventative treatment guidelines. This is not at all surprising when you consider that the average health care provider has 15 minutes in which to hear your complaint, ask you additional questions to complete your medical history, examine you, and review and discuss testing as well as your medications. That 15-minute visit is devoted to assessing all of your health issues. That leaves very little time for lifestyle counseling, prevention advice and addressing your questions. Certainly, neither patients nor insurance companies are willing to pay for additional in-depth counseling from other health care providers, nutritionists or dietitians. If we have a system that is already geared toward not promoting disease prevention and education, what kind of results can we expect?

One answer comes from a recent study called the REACH registry. This study, published in 2006 and one of the largest international studies ever conducted, collected data on almost 68,000 patients worldwide with established atherosclerosis or CHD. This study found that commonly known cardiovascular risk factors like hypertension, diabetes, obesity and elevated cholesterol are largely under-treated and under-controlled in most regions of the world. Even though medical practitioners are well aware of treatment guidelines that establish goals for ideal blood pressure, cholesterol, weight, etc., even in the advanced medical communities of North America and Europe, suboptimal control of these risk factors exists in between 30 percent and 50 percent of all patients receiving medical care. In the less-advanced medical communities of Eastern Europe and Asia, up to 70 percent of all patients who are under the medical care of "qualified" practitioners are not receiving adequate treatment.

> **Alert!** Even in the United States, the Heart and Estrogen/Progesterone Replacement Study (HERS) registry, which followed almost 5,000 women with established CHD, found that only 47 percent were receiving cholesterol-lowering medications. This study and others have repeatedly demonstrated that only 30–50 percent of patients who receive medications to treat the high cholesterol that contributed to their CHD are actually treated to achieve the scientifically validated desirable cholesterol goal that would reduce their risk for future CHD events.

This information clearly indicates that in order for you to make the most of what we know about treating and preventing CHD, you will need to become sufficiently informed to be the advocate for yourself and your family. That is not to say you may not be getting good medical care. You are probably getting the best medical care available within the constraints of our system. It just isn't good enough to do the job of treating and preventing the largest cause of death and disability in the world. Therefore, you simply cannot afford to leave this responsibility solely in the hands of your doctors and other health care providers.

The subsequent chapters will provide a framework for understanding what CHD is and what you can do to prevent it or reverse it. It is my hope that through such understanding, you will become an active participant in your own heart health by adhering to a healthy lifestyle and treatment for CHD. It is also important that you become knowledgeable about the scientific evidence that supports our current guidelines in treating CHD, because only then can you become your own health care advocate and partner with your health care provider to make sure you are receiving the most up-to-date treatment and guidance.

Chapter 2

The Alphabet Soup That Makes Up Heart Disease:
It All Spells Out *Ath-er-o-scle-ro-sis*

MEDICINE, LIKE MOST technical disciplines, has more than its share of abbreviations, acronyms and catchphrases. It is much easier to understand and communicate if we develop a basic knowledge of the vocabulary of heart disease. You have already been introduced to CHD (coronary heart disease). Other abbreviations like MI, CHF, CVD, CVA, TIA, ASCVD, CAD, PVD, PAD, AAA and RAS are all part of the alphabet soup of conditions that are associated with, and/or are a consequence of, atherosclerosis. We will use these terms as we move through the rest of this book. Keep in mind, though, that while each term is a distinct entity, they are all part of the syndrome of atherosclerosis.

What is atherosclerosis? Quite simply, atherosclerosis is the term we use to describe the process by which fat deposits develop inside the arteries of our circulatory system. In fact, the root word *atheroma* means a deposit of fat or, more specifically, an area of lipid plaque.

In this chapter you will gain an understanding of atherosclerosis from both a bird's-eye and a microscopic level. You will see the steps by which arterial plaque develops and perhaps be astounded to learn that the earliest signs of plaque can be detected when we are children. However, before you can understand and appreciate the disease process of atherosclerosis, it is necessary to have a basic understanding of the normal blood circulation system.

Normal Anatomy and Physiology of the Heart and Circulatory System

Our circulatory system consists of 100,000 miles of blood vessels that reach into every organ, muscle and cell in our body. Each minute, over one gallon of blood makes a round-trip circuit through the body to supply all of its tissues with oxygen and nutrients. The first step in the body circuit is oxygen-enriched blood pumping out of the powerful left ventricle, the main pumping chamber of the heart. The blood then enters the main artery in the body, the aorta. It is subsequently delivered to all of the vital organs through the smaller arteries, their branches, the arterioles, and finally the capillaries (**figure 2.1**).

The Blood Circulation Systems: Body and Lung Circuits

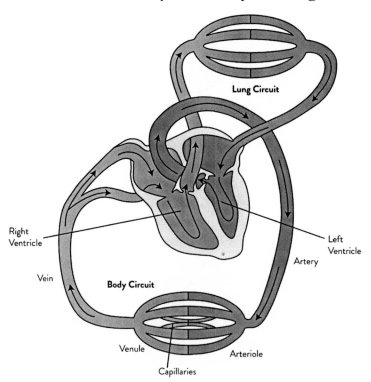

Figure 2.1 Legend: Body Circuit: The blood proceeds from the left ventricle, through the arteries, arterioles, capillary bed, venules, veins and back to the right heart. Lung Circuit: The blood proceeds from the right ventricle, through the lungs and back to the left heart.

Most people believe the blood vessels in the body to be much larger than they actually are. They are, in fact, very small structures. The heart itself is only the size of your fist when clenched tightly. The largest artery in the body is the aorta, which is about the size of a garden hose, measuring no more than one to one-and-a-half inches in diameter. The remaining major arteries of the body are even smaller, typically around one-quarter of an inch in diameter, or about the size of a drinking straw.

The coronary arteries are the blood vessels that drape over the surface of the heart and provide it with its oxygen supply. Arguably, they are the most important arteries in the body. In fact a heart attack, or MI (myocardial infarction), is often called a "coronary." These blood vessels are usually no bigger than a strand of a cooked spaghetti noodle, about one-eighth of an inch in diameter. In fact, they get even smaller as they continue downstream.

The delivery and exchange of oxygen to the tissues of the body occurs at the level of the capillaries. The capillaries are only five to ten microns wide, or about 0.005 inches. A single strand of hair is ten times wider than a single capillary. Capillaries are therefore not visible to the naked eye. They are just large enough to accommodate only one oxygen-containing red blood cell moving in single-file. Every cell in the body is in very close proximity to a capillary. The cells and organs fed by the capillaries extract the oxygen and nutrients from the blood in exchange for carbon dioxide and waste chemicals.

The transit circuit is completed when the now oxygen-poor, carbon-dioxide-enriched blood leaves the capillaries and is transported through the smaller veins, the venules, branch veins, and ultimately the larger veins like the jugular vein and the superior and inferior venae cavae back to the right side of the heart.

The second circuit of blood is the lung circuit, in which the deoxygenated, carbon dioxide-rich blood that has returned from the tissues of the body is pumped from the right side of the heart through the right ventricle to the lungs. Here the carbon dioxide is removed when we exhale and replaced by the oxygen that we inhale through the lung passages. The oxygen-enriched blood then continues into the left side of the heart to be pumped out to the rest of the body and start the circuit once again.

Before we leave the subject of the normal circulation circuit, we will also briefly cover the heart itself. The heart is central to the circulatory system, as it provides the force by which blood is pumped around the circuit of blood vessels. The heart is separated into two distinct compartments, the right side and the left side. The two sides are never in direct communication, even though they are part of the same organ. Each side contains two chambers, the upper chamber, called the atrium, and the lower chamber, called the ventricle. Blood normally flows from the atria to the ventricles and is then pumped out of each ventricle through the squeezing and twisting action of the ventricle. **Figure 2.2** shows the chambers of the heart and the normal route of blood flow.

The Pathway of Blood Flow through the Heart

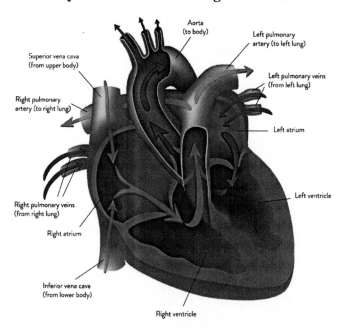

Figure 2.2 Legend: The cardiac chambers, incoming and exiting blood vessels and valves of the heart are shown, with the direction of blood flow indicated by the arrows.

The muscle of the left ventricle is known as the myocardium. It is one of the most powerful muscles in the body, capable of generating more force than any other muscle in the body. The myocardium is stronger than your biceps, quads and hamstrings! It is the action of this muscle that pushes the blood through the entire circuit. The normal function of the myocardium is vital to maintaining good cardiovascular health. In fact the single most important predictor of survival and quality of life for patients with heart disease is how well the myocardium functions and the efficiency with which the left ventricle functions to pump blood.

> **Illumination:** If the muscles of your upper chest were as strong as your heart, you could easily bench-press over 500 pounds! The left ventricle pumps blood with each heart beat, typically 60 times a minute, 24 hours per day, or about two and one-half billion times during your entire life.

Atherosclerosis: A Bird's-Eye View

Now that you understand how normal circulation operates, we can move on to talking about the disease process of atherosclerosis. To appreciate and understand atherosclerosis, you must build up a foundation of knowledge in stages. We will start by introducing you to a bird's-eye view of our circulatory system and the typical places where plaque builds up and causes common clinical problems. The microscopic view of atherosclerosis follows next, when you will see how plaque develops over time inside an artery. This process is typically the same in every artery of the body, whether it is the coronary arteries of the heart, the leg arteries or the cerebral arteries to the brain. Finally, in future chapters, after some background information about cholesterol, we will talk about atherosclerosis at the molecular level. Here you will see the role that cholesterol particles play in the development of arterial plaque. Understanding the molecular basis of plaque formation is important in order to understand the various therapies, diets and supplements that we use to prevent or reverse atherosclerosis.

No organ, tissue or cell in the body can function properly for any length of time without oxygen. As the arteries are the conduits for delivery of oxygen, the buildup of plaque, or atheroma, in these blood vessels is termed atherosclerosis. The term is sometimes used synonymously with *arteriosclerosis*, although technically arteriosclerosis means hardening of the arteries, without necessarily the buildup of plaque. The two processes are so intimately linked that we consider them both as part of the spectrum of cardiovascular disease.

Atherosclerosis can occur in any type of artery. The large arteries that are most often affected are shown in **figure 2.3**. The main artery in the body is the aorta, which runs from the aortic valve as it exits the heart. It makes a 180-degree turn in the upper part of the chest and then travels back down the middle of the chest, through the diaphragm and into the abdomen. There it splits into the right and left iliac arteries, the first branches that begin providing blood to each of the legs. All major arterial branches initially arise from the aorta.

The Heart, Aorta and the Major Arterial Branches

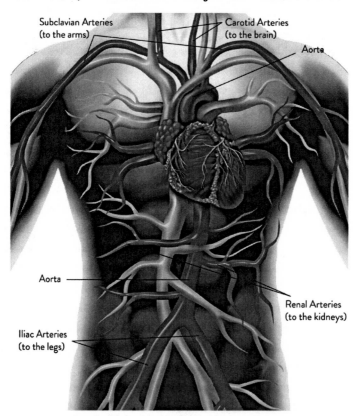

Figure 2.3 Legend: The cardiac chambers, incoming and exiting blood vessels and valves of the heart are shown, with the direction of blood flow indicated by the arrows.

It is noteworthy that the first arterial branches that arise from the aorta are the coronary arteries, the main arterial supply to the heart. The second arterial branches that arise from the aorta are the carotid arteries, which are the main arterial supply to the brain. The significance of the fact that the first blood vessels to originate from the aorta are those providing oxygenated blood flow to the heart and brain should not be lost. Teleologically, the importance of this is obvious: the preservation of blood flow to these two organs, even at the expense of other organs, is absolutely vital. Beyond the origins of the arteries to the heart and the brain, the other arteries then arise, including those to the arms, internal organs of the chest and abdomen, and finally the legs.

When atherosclerosis affects the coronary arteries, it is termed coronary artery disease (CAD) or coronary heart disease (CHD). The terms are interchangeable. CHD can cause a number of heart problems, including angina pectoris, heart attack (also known as a myocardial infarction, or MI), congestive heart failure (CHF), cardiomyopathy, arrhythmias and death.

Arterial Supply of the Heart

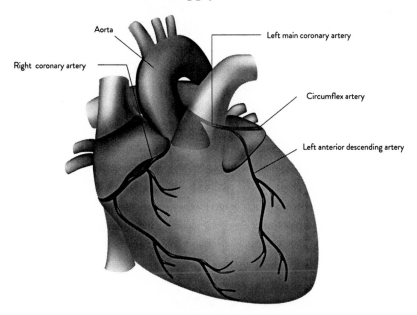

Figure 2.4 Legend: The three major coronary arteries as they run over the surface of the heart are shown.

There are three major coronary arteries (**figure 2.4**), the left anterior descending artery (LAD), the left circumflex artery (LCX) and the right coronary artery (RCA). The LAD and LCX usually arise from a common spot in the aorta, called the left main coronary artery. Each of the three coronary arteries is typically responsible for about one-third of the heart's blood supply. These arteries run over the surface of the heart, like the fingers of one hand draped over a closed fist on the other hand. Atherosclerosis can occur in any or all three of these arteries, as well as in any portion along the length of these arteries. When arteriosclerosis affects a specific spot of an artery, that spot is called a lesion, or stenosis. In many instances, lesions tend to occur in certain spots more than others, such as at bends or branch points of the larger and medium caliber coronary arteries. The development of atherosclerosis in these arteries is responsible for the major clinical syndromes of CHD.

One such syndrome is angina pectoris, or simply angina. Angina is actually the term applied to pain or discomfort that results from the temporary lack of oxygen to the heart when there is an imbalance of oxygen supply and demand. Usually the pain is in the chest, but it can occur in the back, arms or jaw. In some cases, angina may not actually be discomfort, but can manifest itself as shortness of breath, nausea or sweating. In some cases, angina can even be symptomless, or "silent."

The general term for reduced oxygen supply is called ischemia. In most cases, ischemia occurs because plaque narrows the interior opening of the coronary artery, reducing the amount of blood that can flow through. Typically, when there is an increase in the need for oxygen (oxygen demand), such as when you exercise, and that demand is beyond the capability of the heart's coronary arteries to provide adequate blood flow (oxygen supply), the result is the occurrence of ischemia, which manifests itself as chest pain or tightness that is the typical symptom of angina. This mismatch of oxygen supply and demand causing ischemia is in fact the principle behind using stress tests to diagnose CHD.

If there is a more prolonged and total or near-total lack of blood supply to the heart, heart muscle may actually die or malfunction, resulting in a heart attack, or myocardial infarction (MI). This often feels like angina, but it is usually more prolonged or severe. Just as with angina, in many cases heart attacks can also be "silent." When an MI occurs, in many instances the damage to the heart muscle is permanent and irreversible. A large single heart attack or many smaller heart attacks can cause weakening of the heart muscle, resulting in congestive heart failure (CHF) or, if permanent damage exists, a condition called cardiomyopathy. Either temporary lack of oxygen to the heart muscle or scar tissue from permanent heart muscle damage can lead to arrhythmias of the heart, which, if severe enough, can be fatal.

Clinical syndromes resulting from diseases caused by atherosclerosis occur outside the heart also. Atherosclerosis involving the carotid arteries and their branches into the brain is termed carotid artery disease, or cerebrovascular disease (CVD) to signify disease of the brain (cerebral) blood vessels. This plaque buildup can lead to many different syndromes, including a full-blown stroke, or cerebrovascular accident (CVA). Depending on the area of brain deprived of blood and for how long, a CVA can result in paralysis, speech, visual and other sensory problems and even death. In fact not only can a stroke be extremely and permanently disabling, it also often signifies a rapid downward spiral in health, such that the chance of dying within the first year after surviving a stroke is as high as 20 percent.

Another syndrome resulting from cerebrovascular disease is known as a transient ischemic attack (TIA), in which the blood deprivation is temporary and does not result in major damage causing permanent neurological deficits. When the smaller arteries of the brain are involved, more subtle deficits such as memory impairments and even progressive dementia can result.

Outside of the heart and brain, there are a number of other arteries prone to plaque buildup. Plaque buildup in the arteries to the kidneys is termed renal artery stenosis (RAS) and is a common cause of high blood pressure and even kidney failure. When the arteries to the legs are affected, it is called peripheral arterial disease (PAD) or peripheral vascular disease (PVD). This results in an intermittent lack of oxygen to the legs, typically causing pain and cramping in the legs when exertion is attempted, a condition termed claudication. A more profound and constant lack of blood supply to the legs can lead to gangrene that is severe enough to warrant amputation.

Finally, within the aorta itself, atherosclerosis can develop, so that plaque weakens the internal lining of the aorta, causing it to balloon out at the weak points. These weak points most often occur in the abdominal part of the aorta and are called abdominal aortic aneurysms (AAA). However, these weak points can occur in any segment of the aorta and can result in a variety of serious and possibly catastrophic syndromes. If the interior of the aorta narrows, there is restricted blood supply downstream. Sometimes tiny particles of plaque can break loose from the wall of the aorta and migrate downstream, or embolize, resulting in the cutting off of blood supply to other downstream organs and tissues. The bulge from the weakened aorta can put pressure on adjacent organs. An almost universally fatal, but fortunately relatively rare event is a full rupture or burst of the aortic ballooning, or aneurysm.

> **Illumination:** Aortic aneurysms have been the cause of death of several high profile celebrities, among which are George C. Scott, Lucille Ball and John Ritter.

Atherosclerosis: A Microscopic View

The next step in understanding atherosclerosis is to know about the structure of the artery at the microscopic level (**figure 2.5**). The normal artery has three layers. The innermost lining of the artery consists of only one layer of cells and a small underlying band of non-cellular support tissue. This lining is called the *intima* (meaning "inner"), and the cells that compose the lining of the intima are called the *endothelium*. These cells are all tightly connected to one another, creating a barrier to prevent blood from seeping out of the interior of the artery. When healthy, these cells provide a smooth surface on which the blood flows. These cells also have the capability to secrete and respond to various chemicals, hormones and other stimuli. As we will see, a healthy endothelium is critical to preventing atherosclerosis, and, conversely, atherosclerosis does not occur unless the endothelium is diseased. The process of atherosclerosis actually starts just beneath the endothelial cells in the non-cellular tissue of the intima.

The Normal Layers of the Arterial Wall

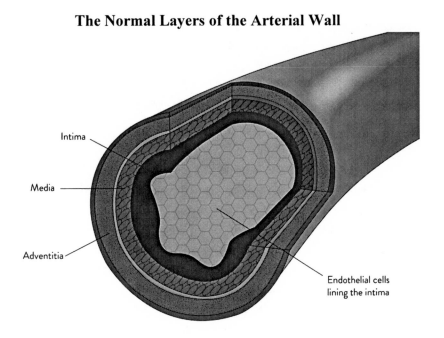

Figure 2.5 Legend: The three layers of the arterial wall: (1) Intima consists of the single-cell layer of cells lining the interior of the artery and the underlying tissue, (2) Media consists of mostly smooth muscle cells, and (3) Adventitia consists of the outermost layer that is made up primarily of supporting tissue.

The middle layer of the artery is called the *media* (meaning "middle"). This layer is a circular ring that surrounds the intima. It is several cells thick and contains mostly muscle cells and other structural and elastic fibers that regulate the tone and size of the artery. The muscle cells respond to stimuli from the adjacent inner layer of endothelial cells, as well as stimuli that they receive from nerves and their own feeder blood vessels, the *vasa vasorum*. These feeder blood vessels penetrate through the outer layers of the artery to provide a blood supply to the cells of the artery itself. In later stages of atherosclerosis, the muscle cells in the medial layer become important participants in the development of plaque.

The outermost layer is called the *adventitia* (meaning "covering layer" of tissue). This layer contains an artery's support system of blood vessels, the vasa vasorum as well as the nerves, and structural fibers of the artery that provide its backbone. This layer also participates in the atherosclerosis process, especially with respect to its involvement with inflammation in the artery.

The Stages of Atherosclerosis

Plaque buildup is a multistage process (**figure 2.6**). It begins with the formation of what is termed a "fatty streak" within the arterial wall. This always requires the deposition or 'laying down' of cholesterol in the wall of the artery. The fatty streak grows silently, without symptoms or warning, and is subject to a variety of influences from cholesterol particles, inflammation and an individual's own genetics. However, even the fatty streak cannot start until the innermost cellular layer of the artery, the endothelium, is damaged. The molecular process by which cholesterol particles enter the arterial wall and cause the fatty streak, as well as the subsequent events in plaque formation will be covered in more detail when we discuss atherosclerosis at the molecular level. What follows below is an overview at the cellular level of the stages of plaque formation.

The fatty streak will evolve into a full-fledged atheroma under the right circumstances. These influences include an abundance of bad cholesterol particles, a lack of good cholesterol particles and the occurrence of inflammation that stimulates protector white blood cells of the body, such as macrophages and T lymphocytes, to attack. Once started, this process continues in a vicious cycle as the body tries to protect itself from the plaque. In fact, the body perceives plaque in the same way as it does a foreign body, and in response lays down more endothelial cells and fibrous tissue in order to isolate and seal off the plaque. The endothelium thickens to form a fibrous capsule or covering, analogous to a scab covering an open skin wound, which causes the blood supply to the plaque to be reduced.

The Progression of Atherosclerotic Plaque

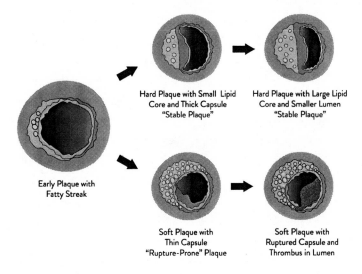

Early Plaque with
Fatty Streak

Hard Plaque with Small Lipid
Core and Thick Capsule
"Stable Plaque"

Hard Plaque with Large Lipid
Core and Smaller Lumen
"Stable Plaque"

Soft Plaque with
Thin Capsule
"Rupture-Prone" Plaque

Soft Plaque with
Ruptured Capsule and
Thrombus in Lumen

Figure 2.6 Legend: The stages of atherosclerosis progressing from the earliest form of plaque called the fatty streak, to mature plaque that may be either soft or hard. Hard plaque is considered stable plaque, but can progress to further narrowing the arterial opening in a slow, gradual manner. Soft plaque is more susceptible to plaque rupture by virtue of its thin capsule, and can lead to hemorrhage, thrombus in the lumen and abrupt occlusion of the artery.

Two additional occurrences further reduce the blood supply to the plaque. The first is the process of inflammation that is occurring in the intima. The second is the smooth muscle cell growth or proliferation occurring on the opposite side of the plaque in the medial and adventitial layers. These processes induce the death of some of the muscle cells and the white blood cells fighting the plaque. The organic material and cholesterol from these dead and dying cells is converted into a weblike matrix that becomes part of the plaque and causes it to grow further. This in turn induces more inflammation and plaque formation, and the entire process continues.

Left unchecked, once the plaque reaches a critical level, for reasons we do not completely understand, the fate of the plaque can follow in one of two directions. In some instances the plaque will grow for years, slowly but steadily, and become hard, like mature scar tissue. This type of plaque usually also develops a thicker fibrous capsule of endothelial cells that cover it and separate it from the blood-containing internal opening of the artery.

Often this type of fibrous plaque contains calcium, the principal element in limestone. In this case, just as in limestone, the plaque is very dense, and is termed "hard" plaque. Initially, the artery adapts to this type of plaque by stretching outward to try to preserve its interior opening for blood to flow. Eventually, though, the plaque starts to protrude inward and cause the opening of the artery to narrow. While this type of plaque can reduce blood supply to the heart, it usually does so quite slowly and typically results in the formation of "stable" plaque. This means it usually is not susceptible to rupture, to distinguish it from the "vulnerable" or "rupture-prone" plaque that will be described below. While stable plaque can cause angina, it does not typically lead to a fatal and sudden heart attack. In fact, only about 30 percent of all heart attacks are caused by this type of "stable" plaque.

Plaque that Progresses to a Heart Attack

The other, more serious fate for plaque is to become "soft" plaque, which is also known as "vulnerable" or "rupture-prone" plaque because it is more susceptible to rupture. The term *rupture* signifies a tearing of the fibrous capsule that overlies the plaque, so that the plaque explodes directly into the artery. Like stable plaque, soft plaque also starts out initially as a fatty streak. Again for reasons we don't completely understand, as soft plaque grows, the layer of endothelial cells that cover the plaque do not form as thick a lining or fibrous capsule as forms with hard plaque. Also, very little calcium enters soft plaque. Since the fibrous capsule that lies on top of this plaque is much thinner, the plaque is much more likely to burst through the endothelial lining.

Often this type of plaque grows even farther toward the outer edge of the artery than "hard" plaque does. Thus, the amount of atheroma may be greater than what is actually contained in the "hard" plaque, but because it does not cause significant narrowing of the interior opening of the artery and impede the flow of blood, there may be no symptoms of reduced blood supply, such as angina. But the increased plaque burden ultimately causes mechanical pressure on the fibrous capsule. This, combined with a high level of inflammation just beneath the surface of the artery, makes it susceptible to rupture.

Continued growth of the "rupture-prone" plaque stretches the fibrous capsule until it gets thinner and thinner. This ticking time bomb is just waiting for an opportunity to erupt and wreak havoc in the artery when the fibrous capsule is punctured. There are many conditions known to provoke rupture of the fibrous capsule. One condition almost universally present is a large degree of inflammation inside the artery. This makes the plaque very active in terms of production of a variety of toxic chemicals as well as attracting aggressive white blood cells like macrophages and T lymphocytes.

The second common condition in plaque rupture is a spike in adrenaline, the hormone that is released when the human body is under stress. This hormone causes blood pressure and pulse to rise and stimulates the release of a variety of other substances that put the body in the "flight or fright" state of readiness. Thus, stresses such as a spike in blood pressure, extreme physical exertion, anger and severe emotional distress can provoke a plaque rupture.

Rupture of soft plaque is the most common cause of an acute heart attack, responsible for over 70 percent of all cases of MI. When plaque ruptures, a whole cascade of harmful events ensues. Blood in the interior of the blood vessel comes into contact with the atheroma, which previously had been sequestered by the fibrous capsule. The exploding plaque, along with all of its toxic chemicals, attracts blood-clotting factors to the site of rupture as the body senses that a blood vessel has been punctured and tries to make a clot at the opening. Within minutes a clot, or thrombus, starts to form. However, instead of sealing off the opening to the plaque, the clot begins to seal off the artery itself, further impairing blood flow. As the blood clot enlarges, the artery may become completely occluded, and oxygen deprivation begins in the muscle downstream that depends on the blood flow through the artery. Within minutes, the metabolism of the downstream cells slows in an effort to stay alive. Continued lack of oxygen ultimately causes the cells to die.

Not only is plaque rupture the most common cause of an acute heart attack, plaque rupture can occur at sites where the amount of plaque and level of obstruction are very small. Typically, we can identify the level of obstruction in an artery by how much of the artery is narrowed by plaque growth. An area of plaque revealed on an angiogram (a picture of the artery obtained using X rays and iodine dye during a catheterization) is considered to be significant if more than 50 percent of the artery is narrowed. Similarly, a stress test will identify only areas of plaque that are large enough to reduce blood flow, again with about 50 percent arterial narrowing.

However, soft and vulnerable plaque occurs more often than not at a level that causes less than 50 percent narrowing of the artery. Therefore, it can be missed by stress tests, and usually is not in an area that is treated with heart stents during a catheterization if it is not causing a problem. Cardiologists are all too familiar with the patient who has a normal stress test one day and the next day is in the emergency room with an acute MI. Even more frightening is the patient who has a "normal" catheterization, only to develop a rupture in an area of plaque several weeks later that was deemed to be "insignificant" during the catheterization.

> **Alert!** Because of the stealthy nature of soft plaque, the goal set by you and your doctor should not be just to treat the plaque that causes the most arterial narrowing, but actually to consider any area of plaque as one that carries a potential to cause a heart attack.

Plaque Formation Starts in Childhood

The multistage process of plaque formation has an extremely variable time-line. The fatty streak can progress to a mature atheroma within as little time as a few months. More typically, the process takes several years. Although all plaque is potentially dangerous, soft or vulnerable plaque is especially concerning. Our understanding about what induces plaque to become either "stable" or "vulnerable" is even more uncertain. However, what we are certain of is that atherosclerosis, CHD and its other manifestations are not an inevitable consequence of just getting older. Heart disease is a lifestyle-borne illness, and the process of atherosclerosis begins in childhood. The scientific evidence for this is overwhelming.

In 1953, an autopsy study of soldiers killed in the Korean War revealed that 77 percent of the hearts examined showed signs of atherosclerosis. The average age of the soldiers was 22 years. These results were confirmed in other studies of Korean and Vietnam War soldiers showing that between 45 percent and 56 percent of the hearts had CHD, and five to six percent had severe narrowing of the coronary arteries. A study from the University of Louisville in Kentucky on victims of noncombat trauma, who had an average age of 26 years, found that 76 percent had CHD, 21 percent had more than 50 percent narrowing of a coronary artery, and nine percent had more than 75 percent narrowing.

The longest and most detailed large-scale study addressing this issue was the Bogalusa Heart Study, begun in 1972 in Bogalusa, Louisiana. Conducted by Tulane University Medical Center in New Orleans, the study examined the hearts of 204 young people between the ages of two and 39 who died in accidents. The study found that 50 percent of the children between the ages of two and 15 years had fatty streaks and that eight percent had full-blown plaque in their coronary arteries. In the older group, between ages 21 and 39, almost all had fatty streaks (85 percent), and 70 percent had CHD. This study and a similar study of nearly 3,000 accident victims called PDAY (Pathobiological Determinants of Atherosclerosis in Youth) both showed that the likelihood of plaque occurrence at a young age was directly related to established risk factors such as physical inactivity, obesity, smoking and high-fat, high-calorie diets.

The evidence that atherosclerosis begins in childhood is incontrovertible. However, that does not mean that the development of CHD is a *fait accompli*. The ongoing growth of plaque is a function of continued exposure to harmful cholesterol particles and a number of other influences that we recognize as cardiovascular risk factors. These include smoking, obesity, high blood pressure and diabetes, to name just a few. As we will see in subsequent chapters, the ability to control and modify these risk factors has a direct impact on not only further development of atherosclerosis, but in the actual ability to reverse atherosclerosis.

Furthermore, the recognition that atherosclerosis begins in childhood should be a major motivator for our society to put a priority on instituting measures to promote healthier lifestyles in our children. The continued increase in childhood obesity, physical inactivity, cigarette smoking and access to high-fat, high-sugar and high-salt diets in our children will only promote an ongoing increase and burden of atherosclerosis in our adult population.

Chapter 3
Cholesterol: The Good, the Bad and the Ugly

AS IMPORTANT AS cholesterol is in the development of Coronary Heart Disease (CHD) and all of the diseases that can result from atherosclerosis, what many people do not realize is that it is also vital to good health. Cholesterol is a naturally occurring steroid molecule that is produced by all mammals. In either the test tube or inside arteries, it looks like a waxy, yellow substance similar to butter. When it is present in high concentrations in the blood, it makes the blood look like cream. When cholesterol is in balance, we stay healthy. When out of balance, the disease process of atherosclerosis takes precedence over the beneficial functions of cholesterol.

This chapter will cover how cholesterol gets into our body and why it is there. We will discuss the various types of lipid particles that carry cholesterol in the bloodstream to the tissues and the arteries of the body. Finally, we will introduce the "lipid hypothesis." This is the concept that forms the basis of our current understanding of how blood cholesterol plays a major role in the development of atherosclerosis.

Cholesterol in Health

Cholesterol is essential for life, as it has a variety of important biological functions. It is an important constituent of cell membranes, where cholesterol both provides structural support and helps regulate the permeability of membranes to allow various substances to pass either in or out of cells.

Cholesterol molecules in the cell membrane are an important constituent of cell receptors. These receptors play a role in cell signaling by facilitating communication and the interaction of cells with their environment. Cholesterol is a major constituent of nerve cells and is important for the proper conduction of nerve impulses. Cholesterol is a necessary precursor in the manufacture of bile acids that are crucial for normal digestion. It is an integral component of steroid hormones, like cortisol and aldosterone, as well as sex hormones, like progesterone, estrogen and testosterone. These hormones regulate a variety of processes involving metabolism, salt and water balance and muscle function, as well as sexual development and function. Finally, cholesterol is a critical component of vitamin D, which is vital to digestion, immunity and good bone health.

There are two sources of cholesterol available to our body. One is called *endogenous*, that which comes from within our body. The liver, primarily, and the intestines, adrenal glands and reproductive organs in our body, to a lesser extent, are all sites of cholesterol synthesis. They collectively make about one gram, equivalent to about one teaspoon, of cholesterol daily. The second source of cholesterol is called *exogenous*, that which comes from the outside. This source is from our diet, through which the average American consumes between 200 and 500 milligrams of cholesterol per day. Thus, more than two-thirds of all the cholesterol in our body comes from tissues in our body that make cholesterol, and less than one-third comes from our diet. From these two sources, the average total cholesterol content that is maintained in our body at any one time is about 35 grams, or about two-thirds of a cup of cholesterol. It is this amount of cholesterol that sits primarily in the tissues of our body and is available for the uses noted above.

Normally, the relative levels of endogenous manufacture and exogenous intake of cholesterol are closely regulated through a process called homeostasis. If cholesterol intake is reduced, endogenous synthesis will increase. Cholesterol is so important and so valuable to the body that it is not wasted. It is recycled for use again in a process known as enterohepatic circulation. Even the cholesterol that ends up in the intestine when excreted in the form of bile salts by the liver to aid digestion is almost all reabsorbed back into the bloodstream from the lower intestinal tract. When there is a disruption in homeostasis, cholesterol can start to play a part in disease.

Cholesterol Metabolism

The pathways for the synthesis of cholesterol are very complex, involving numerous regulatory enzymes, intermediary compounds and feedback signals. In fact, 15 Nobel Prizes have been awarded just for work done in the elucidation of these pathways. However, the brief and simplified overview that follows will provide information that will assist in your understanding of the role cholesterol metabolism plays in atherosclerosis and the rationale for the interventions th`at can prevent or reverse atherosclerosis.

The parent compounds for cholesterol are two organic molecules called acetyl CoA and acetoacetyl CoA. These combine to form the compound 3-hydroxy-3-methylglutaryl coenzyme A, also known as HMG-CoA. This compound is then altered chemically through a process called reduction, with the assistance of the liver enzyme HMG-CoA reductase, to the compound mevalonate. It is important to note that this reduction is irreversible and the most critical step in cholesterol synthesis. This step is also the point of action of statin medications, which are competitive inhibitors, or blockers of the enzyme HMG-CoA reductase.

Not only is the manufacture of cholesterol controlled through the HMG-CoA reductase enzyme, so is the manufacture of mevalonate, squalene and lanosterol, three intermediary compounds that are formed before the final cholesterol molecule is generated. All of these compounds also have important biological functions. These downstream steps also require the energy compound adenosine tri-phosphate, also known as ATP. It is believed that many of the side effects of statins are caused by either depletion of these other compounds or effects on ATP, or very rarely by a reduction in cholesterol itself so that it is not available for its normal biological functions.

As complex as the pathway for the manufacture of cholesterol is, the homeostatic mechanisms for maintaining optimal cholesterol levels are even more elegant and intricate. One of the most important of these mechanisms is the process regulating how cholesterol is added and removed from the bloodstream. One important family of proteins residing inside cells that help to regulate cholesterol homeostasis is the group called sterol regulatory element-binding proteins (SREBP). The SREBPs act directly upon DNA to affect the transcription of genes that control the manufacture and metabolism of cholesterol. The activity and amount of HMG-CoA reductase is regulated through these actions of SREBPs. Also affected by the SREBPs is the activity and manufacture of the surface liver receptors and other cellular receptors for "bad" cholesterol, known as the LDL receptor. The actions of this receptor largely control the removal of cholesterol from the bloodstream. Although their primary effect is on HMG-CoA reductase, the main mechanism by which statins lower cholesterol is through an increase in the activity of the LDL receptor.

Lipoproteins: The Constant Companions of Cholesterol

Cholesterol is a fatty, oily substance. It is termed *hydrophobic*, from the Greek, meaning "fearful of water," to signify that it is only slightly soluble in water. Our body is of course 60–70 percent water, and our bloodstream is almost all water. How can cholesterol function in this type of environment? The answer is that cholesterol is almost never found in the body by itself. To make cholesterol soluble so that it dissolves in the bloodstream and in the watery milieu inside cells, it is attached and incorporated into particles or clusters of fat called lipid particles. The word lipid is also derived from the Greek, in this case the word *lipos*, meaning "fat." Since the fat portion is combined with a protein component, the proper descriptor for these particles is *lipoproteins*.

Lipoproteins are complex disk-shaped particles that can be thought of as jelly-filled doughnuts (**figure 3.1**). The outer layer, or the dough, is *hydrophilic*, from the Greek for "loving of water." This layer is composed of proteins called apolipoproteins. The outer layer also contains water-friendly lipid particles called phospholipids and some free cholesterol that is wrenched among the phospholipid particles. The inner core, or jelly, is where all of the hydrophobic fats are located, including most of the cholesterol and the other major fat particles, triglycerides.

In addition to providing a soluble means for transporting cholesterol through the blood, lipoproteins have cell-targeting signals that direct the lipids to certain tissues. The apolipoproteins on the surface of the lipoprotein molecules are the primary regulators that determine the fate,

Model of a lipoprotein particle

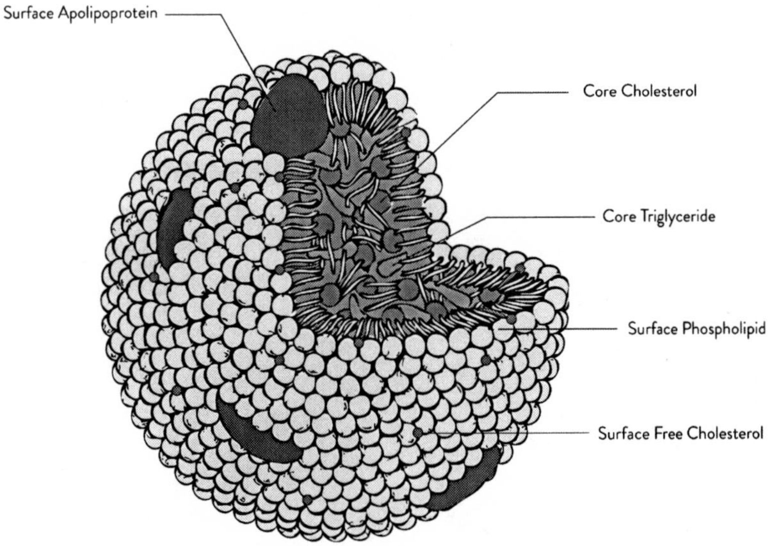

Figure 3.1 Legend: All lipoprotein particles consists of an outer hydrophilic layer composed of surface apolipoproteins, phospholipids and some free cholesterol, and an inner hydrophobic core composed of the fatty substances, cholesterol and triglycerides.

function and destination of the lipoproteins. These surface apolipoproteins function through their chemical composition and geometric conformation to act as surface homing devices that direct the entire lipoprotein particle to its intended destination. Furthermore, once at their programmed destination, the apolipoproteins facilitate the transfer of cholesterol between their lipoprotein particles and the cells for which they are targeted by interacting and binding with the specific receptors on the cells.

Lipoproteins are classified into five major groups, according to their size and density (**figure 3.2**). The largest and lightest, or least dense, are the chylomicrons. These particles are less dense than water (density 0.93 gm/mL, compared to water's density of 1 gm/mL), so in a test tube they would float on top of water. They are quite variable in size, ranging from 75 to 1,200 nanometers (one nm is one millionth of a centimeter) in diameter. The largest chylomicron is therefore actually quite large, as it would be about one-fifth the size of a single red blood cell. After chylomicrons, in order of decreasing size and increasing density are the Very Low Density Lipoproteins (VLDL), Intermediate Density Lipoproteins (IDL), Low Density Lipoproteins (LDL) and, finally, the High Density Lipoproteins (HDL).

Lipoprotein classes organized by size and density

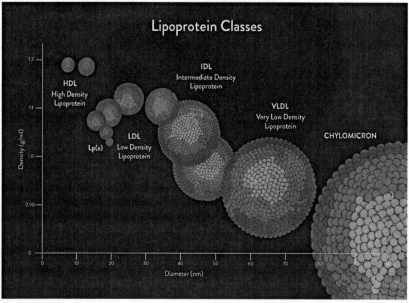

Figure 3.2 Legend: The five major lipoprotein classes can be distinguished by the size and density of the lipoprotein particles. The largest and least dense are the chylomicrons, followed by the VLDL, IDL, LDL and finally the smallest and most dense particles, the HDL.

As we will see later, VLDL, IDL and LDL particles are the atherogenic particles since they promote the development of atherosclerosis. Of these, the most important is LDL, which we commonly think of as "bad" cholesterol. Conversely, HDL is anti-atherogenic as it is responsible for removal of cholesterol from the bloodstream, and is the particle that is commonly known as "good" cholesterol.

In general, more fat relative to protein content in a lipoprotein corresponds to lower density. So the chylomicrons and VLDL particles have more fat content than do the HDL particles. The type of cholesterol that is within each of the classes of lipoproteins is all chemically identical. Thus, it is not the type of cholesterol that makes the particle a good or bad lipo-protein, but rather the amount of cholesterol relative to the non-cholesterol components as well as the surface apolipoproteins, that determines how that particular particle will function.

Chylomicrons are involved primarily in the exogenous pathway for cholesterol metabolism. They develop in the bloodstream after dietary fat is absorbed through the small intestine in the form of small bubbles called micelles. The micelles are similar to the bubbles you see when you vigor-ously shake a bottle of oil and vinegar salad dressing. The absorption of this fat requires the activity of enzymes in the intestinal lining. When these enzymes are deficient or not working, fat absorption is blocked. One such important enzyme is called the Niemann-Pick C1-like protein, which is a target for some cholesterol-lowering medications.

Chylomicrons are the main transporters of fats absorbed in digestion from the intestine for delivery to muscle and other tissues. Chylomicrons consist mostly of free fatty acids combined with compounds called glycerols that combine to form triglycerides. The main fat particles in chylomicrons are in fact triglycerides and not cholesterol. The cholesterol that is within chylomicrons is mostly hydrophobic and resides within the core. The pri-mary apolipoprotein in chylomicrons is called Apo B48. The lipid compo-nents of chylomicrons are used for energy or fat production. As the chylomicrons circulate in the bloodstream, various cells remove some of their lipid components, especially the triglycerides. The cholesterol that remains in the more cholesterol-rich chylomicrons that are now formed is either stored in fat cells for later use or taken up from the bloodstream by the liver for metabolic needs.

Atherogenic Lipoproteins. Atherogenic lipoproteins are the lipid particles that promote plaque development. Chylomicrons are typically not atherogenic. The chylomicrons formed in the small intestine eventually reach the liver. It is there that the VLDL and IDL molecules are produced from what remains of the fatty acids in the chylomicrons and from the cholesterol that is not used by the liver to make bile salts. This process is the beginning of the endogenous pathway of cholesterol metabolism. It is also here that the Apo B48 chylomicron surface apolipoprotein is converted to the Apo B100 apolipoprotein. The VLDL and IDL molecules contain

Apo B100 as their main apolipoprotein. As we will see, the Apo B100 molecule is what confers the property of atherogenicity to a lipid particle.

As the VLDL and IDL particles go through the bloodstream, various lipid components are removed, depending on the needs of the tissues that are supplied. VLDLs and most IDLs are present in the bloodstream for only a very short time, typically no more than 30–60 minutes. The activity of bloodstream enzymes and the tissues that extract lipid components from these particles quickly changes these VLDLs and IDLs to even more cholesterol and protein-rich, denser particles.

As this process continues, the VLDLs and IDLs are transformed into the most cholesterol-rich particles, LDL particles. The typical LDL particle contains no more than 10 percent triglyceride and is 90 percent or more cholesterol. However, in a milieu that is high in triglycerides, LDLs can absorb more triglyceride.

LDL particles are the major bloodstream carriers of cholesterol and are commonly known as "bad" cholesterol. Unlike VLDL and IDL particles, which remain in the bloodstream for only a few hours, LDLs can linger for two to three days. This makes more LDL available to the cells of the body requiring cholesterol. It also makes LDL more available for atherosclerosis.

The outer shell of each LDL contains just one molecule of the apolipoprotein Apo B100. The surface-bound Apo B100 serves as a signal to tissues that contain the LDL receptor to attract and bind the entire LDL complex. After binding to the cell surface, the entire LDL lipoprotein molecule is ingested through the membrane of the cell, and once it is inside the cytoplasm of the cell, the cholesterol is extracted and used for whatever the cell needs.

The LDL receptor on the surface of cells is vital for not only the health of the cell, but also in determining how much cholesterol is free to circulate in the bloodstream. When there is a relative deficiency of LDL receptors, or abnormal function of LDL receptors, excess LDL molecules appear in the blood. These particles then become available to blood vessels for the process of atherosclerosis.

Atheroprotective Lipoproteins. The most dense lipoprotein particle is HDL. It is the only lipid particle known to retard plaque development. It is thus considered atheroprotective. Like all other lipoproteins except chylomicrons, HDLs are also initially made mostly in the liver, and to a lesser extent in the intestinal cells. They are very similar to the other lipoproteins in their basic structure. However, they differ from other lipoproteins in a very important way. The HDL surface apolipoprotein is Apo A.

By virtue of the unique properties of the Apo A molecule attached to the surface, HDL particles do not deliver cholesterol to cells or arteries. Instead, HDL particles function primarily to transport cholesterol back to the liver for excretion or to other tissues that use cholesterol for synthesis. This process is known as reverse cholesterol transport. HDLs may also have protective properties that are unrelated to their role in cholesterol metabolism. Thus, HDL is known as "good" cholesterol. Large numbers of HDL particles that function normally are associated with better health outcomes due to a reduced risk of atherosclerosis.

HDL particles promote the removal of cholesterol from cells in several ways. However, the primary mechanism by which this occurs is that HDL particles attach to the surface of cells. The Apo A on these particles uniquely confers upon them the ability to promote the transfer of cholesterol from within the cell to the surface of the cell and ultimately to the HDL particle. This process requires the HDL to interact with special ATP-binding cassette transporter proteins in the cell membrane. For the purposes of classification, these proteins have been given names such as ABC A1, ABC G1 and ABC G4.

After the cholesterol is transferred from a cell to the HDL particle, the HDL can rid itself of cholesterol in several ways. One way is through the direct method, in which it is carried to the cholesterol-generating organs, such as the liver, adrenal glands, testes and ovaries. These organs contain "scavenger" receptors for HDL on their surfaces. The main scavenger receptor is known by the name SR B1. These surface receptors bind the circulating HDL, causing the particles to dock at the site of Apo A, in the same way as a spaceship docks at a space station. Once the HDL particle is docked, the cholesterol inside is extracted, and the HDL particle is released back into the circulation in order to go out to retrieve and transport more cholesterol. The extracted cholesterol is metabolized by the organ or, if in the liver, it can be excreted as bile salts.

The second fate of cholesterol retrieved by HDL particles is in the blood circulation itself. This is called the indirect pathway, which is mediated by an enzyme called cholesterol ester transfer protein (CETP). This enzyme facilitates the exchange and transfer of triglycerides from VLDL particles for cholesterol from HDL particles. In this process, by receiving additional cholesterol, the VLDL is converted to LDL, which can then be removed by LDL receptors, primarily in the liver. The triglycerides that transfer back to the HDL are unstable in the circulation and are quickly degraded by blood enzymes, leaving the HDL particle behind to restart the process of retrieving and transporting cholesterol. The CETP enzyme is of special interest, as new medications that inhibit CETP are currently being developed. Early studies indicate these may be very potent therapies to both raise HDL and lower LDL.

There is abundant evidence that having high levels of well-functioning HDL is protective against atherosclerosis. Conversely, one of the most important risk factors of MI, stroke, CHD, and PVD is a low level of HDL cholesterol. Although it is believed that the main protective function of HDLs is to remove cholesterol from the arterial wall, HDLs have been shown to enhance good cardiovascular health and reduce the risk of CHD through other mechanisms also. These mechanisms include antioxidant, anti-inflammatory, anti-clotting and endothelial cell repair effects.

Cholesterol in Disease: The Lipid Hypothesis

Cholesterol was first identified as a constituent of human atherosclerotic plaque only 100 years ago, in 1910, by the Nobel Prize-winning chemist Adolf Windhaus. Soon thereafter, two Russian physicians, Nikolay Anichkov and Semen Chalatov, demonstrated that rabbits who were fed large quantities of cholesterol developed atherosclerotic plaque. Through these observations, the notion that high levels of cholesterol in the bloodstream caused the development of atherosclerosis or the "lipid hypothesis" was born.

Two large observational trials provided further support for the premise that abnormal cholesterol levels were associated with CHD. The Seven Countries Study during the 1950s and 1960s established the association between dietary fat consumption and abnormal blood lipids and risk of heart disease. The other major trial was the Framingham Heart Study, started in 1948 in the working-class community of Framingham, Massachusetts, which has been a robust source of epidemiological data on CHD and lipids. In fact, the study continues to collect data even today. One of the first observations in the Framingham study, published in 1961, showed that in a cohort of 4,000 men and women, high blood pressure, smoking and high blood cholesterol were preventable factors contributing to the development of heart disease.

The transformation from hypothesis to accepted fact was first realized in 1984, when the Lipid Research Clinics Coronary Primary Prevention Trial (LRC-CPPT) was published. In this study, almost 4,000 men with high cholesterol, but without any evidence of CHD, were treated with cholestyramine as a cholesterol-lowering therapy. Cholestyramine was one of the earliest fat blockers developed that prevented the intestinal absorption of dietary fat. Although it is not used very much now because it is very poorly tolerated due to intestinal side effects and because better therapies are available, subjects who took this drug reduced their cholesterol by an average of nine percent and their LDL cholesterol by 12 percent. This corresponded with a 19 percent lower risk of having CHD events over the next seven years.

This trial led to the development of a change in public health policy regarding cholesterol in the United States and throughout the world. The National Cholesterol Education Program (NCEP) was born. This led to the "know your cholesterol, know your risk" initiative that encouraged all Americans to get their cholesterol checked, and provided guidance on optimal levels of cholesterol. The NCEP continues today. It has gone through several updates to reflect the current state of knowledge about lipid disorders and how they should be managed. As we will see in subsequent chapters, the NCEP is one of the main sources of guidelines to health care providers for treating cholesterol and lipid disorders.

Chapter 4
Atherosclerosis, More Than Just Clogged Pipes:
Cellular and Molecular Mechanisms of Plaque Buildup

THE CLOSER WE examine the process of atherosclerosis the more complex it appears. The common misperception is that atherosclerosis is simply a clogging of the artery by cholesterol, in the same way as the drain from your sink clogs up from years of kitchen debris being tossed into it. The simplistic explanation for the cure then lies in the hope that we will someday develop a Drano for our arterial pipes, and magically the disease will disappear. Sadly, the perception of the disease and cure are far from what actually occurs.

There is no doubt that atherosclerosis is primarily a disease caused by cholesterol deposition in the arterial wall. We have already learned that this is a dynamic process with both addition and removal of cholesterol ongoing continuously. In order for plaque to grow, the amount of cholesterol deposited must be in excess of the amount that is removed. However, there are a number of other factors involved in the accumulation of cholesterol plaque. The body has various mechanisms to protect us against atherosclerosis. In some cases these mechanisms work well and play a beneficial role. But in some instances these mechanisms are actually counterproductive or maladaptive.

In this chapter we will look at the development of plaque at the cellular and molecular levels. This will include an examination of how cholesterol deposits occur in the arterial wall. We will discuss in detail the roles of LDL, HDL and other lipid particles that are involved in the atherosclerosis process. You will also see that in addition to cholesterol deposition, three additional processes occur in the arterial wall that affects the development and fate of plaque: endothelial dysfunction, vascular inflammation and arterial thrombosis. These factors are all interrelated and influence each other to both enhance and mitigate the atherosclerosis process. From this understanding, you will see that instead of a magical Drano, the cure for atherosclerosis is to attack it on the fronts of all the processes that facilitate its development.

Endothelial Dysfunction

You will recall from Chapter two that the endothelium is the artery's inner wallpaper, consisting of only a single cell layer, which lines the blood vessels and separates the blood from the internal layers of the arteries. The endothelium functions to protect the wall of the artery in the same way as your skin protects the tissues underneath it. One sign of the importance of the endothelium as a protective barrier is the sheer size of the endothelium. Whereas the surface area of the skin in humans is about one and one-half to two square meters, the surface area of endothelium in humans is between 4,000 and 7,000 square meters.

> **Illumination:** If lined up end-to-end, the endothelial cells from a single person would wrap more than four times around the circumference of the Earth.

When endothelial cells no longer function properly, a condition known as endothelial dysfunction results. Endothelial dysfunction is the earliest sign that a region of an artery is prone to atherosclerosis. In fact, without endothelial dysfunction, plaque development can neither start nor continue. Endothelial cells have a variety of regulating functions related to maintaining blood vessel tone, preventing blood clotting and both facilitating and preventing the absorption of a variety of substances in the bloodstream into the wall of the blood vessel. When these functions are adversely affected, the endothelium can no longer protect the arterial wall.

The endothelium is susceptible to damage from a variety of factors. Mechanical stress on the endothelium in the form of shear forces caused by perturbations in blood flow at branch points or bends in the blood vessel is a common cause of endothelial dysfunction. This is why plaque often develops in these spots in arteries. Elevated blood pressure can also put stress on the endothelium. Blood pressure is the mechanical pressure applied to the walls of the artery. Since the blood is in direct contact with the endothelium, this layer of cells is most directly affected by elevations in blood pressure. Elevated blood lipids, blood sugar, and adrenaline levels, chemicals from tobacco smoke, and a variety of other chemicals and influences create stress on the endothelium. All of these factors are associated with chronic and continuous endothelial damage. In some cases, these stresses can also suddenly damage the endothelium, as in the case of a rupture of the fibrous capsule that overlies an area of plaque, and cause an acute heart attack or stroke.

When the endothelium is subject to such stress, it can no longer function as a barrier to prevent harmful substances in the bloodstream from entering into the wall of the artery. This loss of function can occur when the junctions between the endothelial cells develop small gaps that physically permit substances in the bloodstream to seep into the wall of the artery beneath the endothelium. By another mechanism, the endothelial cells themselves can malfunction with respect to their ability to block the entry of substances through their membranes. When this happens, a variety of harmful and plaque-promoting chemicals and cells gain access to the tissues of the arterial wall beneath the endothelium. Lastly, malfunctioning endothelial cells lose their ability to trigger the chemical reactions that cause the relaxation and constriction of their blood vessels. This function, called vasoreactivity, is necessary for altering the caliber of the artery lined by the endothelium. Vasoreactivity is very important in regulating blood flow inside the lumen of the artery as well as chemical processes inside the wall of the artery.

The Role of LDL in Cholesterol Deposition

Although we think of cholesterol and arterial plaque as if they were synonymous, in fact, one's level of Total Cholesterol is of almost no value in assessing one's risk for Coronary Heart Disease (CHD). Data from the Framingham Heart Study (discussed in Chapter three) conclusively showed that blood levels of Total Cholesterol are in fact not very different between people who do and people who do not have CHD. At first glance, this may seem like a contradiction to the concept of the lipid hypothesis that we discussed earlier. However, what this observation indicates is that atherosclerosis is much more complex than simply an elevation in blood cholesterol. As we will see, various cholesterol particles and features of the arterial endothelium, inflammation and thrombosis play a major role in the development of atherosclerosis and the clinical syndromes that result.

Much more so than Total Cholesterol, scientific evidence indicates that the lipoprotein LDL is central to the development of plaque and the clinical syndromes that occur with atherosclerosis. As we have already discussed, LDL is a cholesterol-rich particle that carries one molecule of the apolipoprotein Apo B100 on its surface. This particle is especially prone to depositing its cholesterol into the walls of arteries. In particular, the Apo B100 appears to act as a magnet on the LDL particle for the endothelial cells that line the insides of arteries.

"LDL-C" is the abbreviation for the measured amount of cholesterol (the "-C" designation) inside the core of the LDL particle itself. When your cholesterol levels are tested, the LDL-C number that is reported is your bad cholesterol. Specific target ranges for LDL-C are determined by your unique medical issues and risk factors.

The primary carrier of cholesterol for delivery to the artery is the LDL particle. As is the case for endothelial dysfunction, an abnormal level of LDL-C is a necessary, albeit not always sufficient, condition for atherogenesis. As you will see, these processes operate together and in concert.

> **Illumination:** For most people LDL-C should be below 160 mg/dL. It should be much lower if you already have or are at a high risk for developing CHD. The NCEP guidelines help determine optimal LDL-C levels based upon an individual's CHD risk.

LDL particles circulate freely in the bloodstream, and actually roll over the surface of the endothelium, just like bowling balls rolling down an alley. If the endothelium is damaged, LDL particles can gain access to the tissue that lies in the arterial wall beneath the endothelium. The Apo B100 molecule that is on the surface of each LDL particle (and most VLDL and IDL particles also) has the ability to bind to various proteins and structural components that normally reside just beneath the endothelium within the intimal layer of the artery. In this way LDL cholesterol is retained or trapped inside the vessel wall. Once inside the wall of the artery, the LDL is subject to the chemical process of oxidation. This process is particularly injurious to the arterial wall and has several consequences. As might be expected, the more LDL particles, Apo B100 and LDL-C, the greater the risk of atherosclerosis, as more particles are available to enter the arterial wall, to be oxidized and to be retained for plaque formation (**figure 4.1**).

When oxidation of an LDL particle occurs, the body senses the event as an injury caused by an invader inside the artery. These signals emanate from the endothelial cells themselves, as the process of oxidation causes these cells to become "activated." In this activated state, these cells undergo a variety of chemical and structural changes. One of the most important is that they sprout chemical adhesion molecules, also known as CAMs, on their surface membranes. These molecules act like Velcro or flypaper, and make the normally smooth and lubricated arterial wall sticky. The CAMs attract even more LDL particles and also facilitate the binding of endothelial cells to a variety of white blood cells in the bloodstream that are involved in inflammation, the most important of which are monocytes and lymphocytes. The white blood cells so attracted also find the small gaps between the dysfunctional endothelial cell junctions, and enter the intima.

Schematic of lipoprotein particles moving through the bloodstream

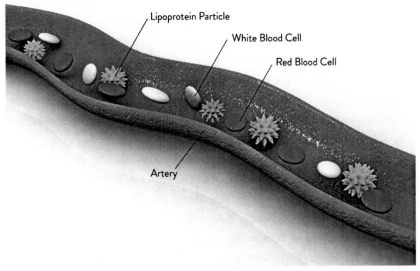

Figure 4.1 Legend: Lipoproteins transport cholesterol and triglycerides through the bloodstream. When they come in close contact with the endothelial lining of the artery, they can interact with the endothelial cells as well as the tissue in the arterial wall.

With the white blood cells, the stimulated immune system mounts a counterattack against the oxidized LDL. Inflammatory cells are attracted specifically to the area of oxidized LDL in the intima. The monocytes in particular are stimulated to transform into killer inflammatory cells called macrophages. *Macrophage* literally means "big eater," and like the Pac-Man icon in the video game, these macrophages gobble up the activated or oxidized LDL particles. Once the macrophages become full of LDL cholesterol particles they transform into foam cells, so termed because under a microscope the fat particles inside make the cells look as if they are filled with foamy bubbles. The foam cells are the building blocks of cholesterol plaque, and a cluster of foam cells is what constitutes a fatty streak. You will recall from our earlier discussion that the fatty streak is the first precursor of atherosclerotic plaque.

As lipids continue to accumulate, the macrophages and foam cells are stimulated to express LDL receptors on their surfaces. This is a maladaptive process, because it further stimulates the uptake of oxidized LDL and LDL cholesterol. This can further trigger the entry of other inflammatory cells into the area. The continued increase in foam cells and lipid accumulation causes the intimal layer of the artery to thicken. This process reduces the diffusion of oxygen from the blood through all of the layers in the wall of the blood vessel. As the oxygen supply diminishes, the cells in the intimal layer of the artery begin to die, a process called apoptosis. The death of these cells causes the release of their internal components, which create a gelatinous matrix in this layer of the artery that, along with cholesterol, is a primary constituent of plaque.

The death of cells in the intima also stimulates the entry of muscle cells from the middle or medial layer of the artery to enter the intima. These cells are normally sequestered in the medial layer by a thin membrane that separates them from the intima. When stimulated to migrate into the intima by the development of plaque, they enhance plaque growth in several ways. They can act like foam cells and absorb cholesterol. They also make collagen, a structural protein that provides a platform on which plaque can grow. Another response to plaque development is new blood vessel growth from the outermost layer of the artery, the adventitia. These blood vessels help to fuel the fire of inflammation and cholesterol delivery. All of these processes continue in a dynamic and simultaneous manner.

As shown in **figure 4.2**, these processes result in a self-generating, vicious cycle. The endothelial damage permits LDL cholesterol particles to penetrate into the arterial wall. The LDL particles are trapped and retained in the web-like mixture of molecular proteins and sugars that reside in the intimal layer of the artery, called the proteoglycan matrix. Once trapped, the LDL particles are oxidized, stimulating an inflammatory response. The uptake of oxidized LDL particles into macrophages results in the formation of foam cells. These cells coalesce to form the cellular components of atherosclerotic plaque. The plaque growth results in oxygen deprivation to the inflammatory and foam cells, resulting in cell death (apoptosis). The debris from dying cells adds non-cellular components into the plaque. This causes more endothelial dysfunction and the entry of more LDL particles, perpetuating the cycle.

Incorporation of the LDL particle into lipid plaque

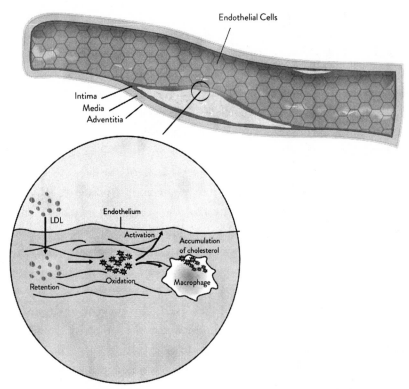

Figure 4.2 Legend: The process by which bloodstream LDL particles enter the arterial wall through the endothelial cells, are retained and then transformed into oxidized particles and subsequently consumed by macrophages to form the first elements of lipid plaque is shown.

As the plaque grows, the artery initially adapts by enlarging at its outermost boundary, so that the plaque grows toward the outer edge of the artery. In this way, the interior opening of the artery is maintained, permitting blood to continue to pass without obstruction. Several other adaptations to plaque growth occur inside the arterial wall. One is that the endothelium of the artery thickens in the area immediately adjacent to the plaque, forming a fibrous capsule of cells that helps to mechanically contain the plaque. The other adaptation is that calcium is induced to enter the plaque. One of the hardest minerals in the body, calcium forms crystals or spicules that weave through the plaque. These calcium deposits help to stabilize the plaque in the same way that re-bars reinforce concrete.

The Role of HDL in Cholesterol Removal

HDL is a lipoprotein particle that, as we learned in the last chapter, is primarily involved in reverse cholesterol transport. It is also a dynamic player in the plaque formation process. Within plaque, HDL facilitates the active removal of cholesterol. By binding to the macrophages that have entered the intima through its Apo A docking port, the HDL particle helps to remove cholesterol from within these cells. The HDL particle then reenters the bloodstream and delivers the cholesterol back to the liver. Thus, HDL functions as the garbage truck for hauling cholesterol. HDL does a curbside pickup of excess cholesterol within the cell and transports it through the bloodstream back to the dumping site for cholesterol, the liver.

In addition to promoting the active removal of cholesterol, HDL also plays a number of other roles that retard the generation of plaque. It can enhance endothelial function and retard plaque growth through its anti-inflammatory and antioxidant properties. HDL prevents accumulation of cholesterol in the intima by hydrolyzing oxidized LDL. This process essentially reverses the oxidation of LDL particles and so makes them less susceptible to absorption into macrophages. HDL also prevents inflammatory responses and reduces monocyte infiltration into the intima by the effect it has of decreasing CAM expression in endothelial cells.

HDL's anti-inflammatory effects not only retard plaque growth and development but also help to restore normal endothelial function. These effects appear to be a significant influence in keeping plaque in a stable state rather than letting it become vulnerable to the point where it is likely to rupture. These properties of HDL help to explain why high levels of HDL are associated with a lower risk of atherosclerosis. They also help to explain why high levels of HDL appear to be associated with a reduced risk of the sudden illnesses that occur from abrupt plaque rupture, such as heart attack and stroke.

The Role of Lipoprotein Particle Subtypes in Atherosclerosis

The five major lipoproteins discussed in Chapter three can be further classified by additional subtypes of particles. As shown in **figure 3.2**, these subtypes also differ from each other in their size and density. Some of these particle subtypes, through seemingly minor alterations in their chemical composition or structure, become important facilitators of the process of atherosclerosis.

LDL. Within the category of LDL particles, one subtype of particle is larger and, based on its lipid composition, less dense than other LDL particles. This type is called large, buoyant LDL. On the other end of the spectrum are the smaller and denser LDL particles. In most cases, in a dynamic process, an individual LDL particle continuously changes size and density as various lipid components are added or depleted.

The small, dense LDL particles have easier access to enter the arterial wall. Imagine the small, dense LDL particles as heavy bowling balls. A heavier and smaller bowling ball can more easily traverse the junctions between the endothelial cells. Once the small, dense LDL particles enter the intimal layer of the artery, they are also more easily trapped in the proteoglycan matrix and oxidized. The large, buoyant LDL particles are like beach balls. Too large to pass through the endothelial junctions, they harmlessly float and bounce through the bloodstream, never penetrating the endothelial cell wall into the lining of the artery (**figure 4.3**).

Small and Large LDL Particles

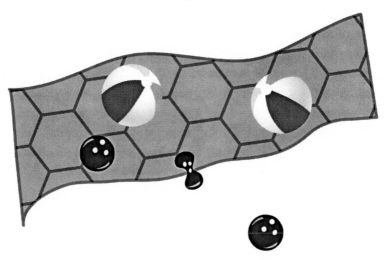

Figure 4.3 Legend: Smaller LDL particles, like bowling balls, can more easily penetrate through the endothelial cell lining barrier of the artery to enter the arterial wall. The larger LDL particles, like beach balls, harmlessly float in the bloodstream.

The corollary to the concept of varying atherogenicity of LDL particles based upon their size and density is that when there is a preponderance of small, dense LDL particles, there is also an increase in the number of LDL particles. This is simply a result of conservation of mass. Imagine that if we shatter a big single stone with a hammer, we will be left with lots of little stones. In the same way, if a larger LDL particle is converted into smaller particles, there must be more particles. However, in order to maintain their unique identity as LDL, both the small, dense and the large, buoyant types of LDL each contain exactly one Apo B100 surface apolipoprotein molecule. So when there is a preponderance of small, dense LDL particles, there are more atherogenic Apo B100 molecules also.

A number of factors affect the proportion of LDL particles of a specific size and density. One common condition is when blood triglyceride levels are high, and the LDL particles incorporate more triglycerides into their structure. This effectively works like a hammer, causing the LDL particles to break up into more numerous, smaller and denser LDL particles.

When there is an increase in the number of small, dense LDL particles, the amount of measurable LDL-C may not change. Yet an environment of more small, dense LDL particles is much more atherogenic. How is this possible? The answer is that for the purposes of plaque formation, the number of Apo B100-containing particles is much more important than the amount of cholesterol these particles contain.

Consider the analogy of LDL particles as automobiles on a highway. The passengers inside the automobiles represent the amount of cholesterol carried by each particle. The occurrence of a traffic jam depends on how many cars are present on the highway much more so than how many passengers are being carried. In the same way, having more Apo B100-containing LDL particles is much worse than having more LDL-C (**figure 4.4**).

This is one explanation for why there is more to determining cardiovascular risk than just LDL-C levels. No doubt LDL-C is important, but perhaps at least equally important is the number of LDL particles. This number can actually be measured by advanced lipid testing methods, as we will discuss in Chapter seven. The number of Apo B100 molecules directly reflects the number of LDL particles, since there is always one molecule of

Apo B100 with each LDL particle. Therefore, measurement of Apo B100 is also useful. The distribution of the type of LDL particles in terms of their density can also be measured. Generally, the risk of atherosclerosis is increased as the proportion of small, dense LDL particles is increased.

LDL-Particle Number versus LDL-Cholesterol

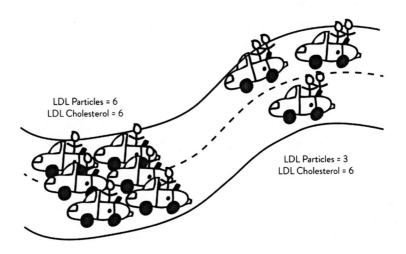

LDL Particles = 6
LDL Cholesterol = 6

LDL Particles = 3
LDL Cholesterol = 6

Figure 4.4 Legend: In this example, both sets of cars have the same number of passengers (LDL cholesterol=6). However, there are more cars (LDL particles) in the left panel (LDL particles =6) than the right (LDL particles = 3), so there is more clogging of the highway artery in the left panel. Since the cars carry the passengers, in the same way as LDL particles carry the cholesterol, atherosclerosis is more likely to occur with a higher LDL particle number than a higher LDL-cholesterol content.

LDL is, of course, not the only particle playing a role in atherosclerosis. The other lipoproteins, including the triglyceride-rich chylomicrons, VLDL, and IDL, can also promote a milieu that promotes atherosclerosis. This typically occurs when the level of these particles is sufficiently elevated that either more cholesterol is made available to be incorporated into the LDL particles, or more LDL particles are actually made. In fact VLDL and IDL also contain one molecule of Apo B100. There is good statistical evidence that supports the premise that total Apo B100 levels correlate more with risk of atherosclerosis than do any measurements of total cholesterol or LDL-C.

Lipoprotein (a). An additional lipoprotein particle that is worthy of mention is called lipoprotein (a), or Lp(a). This molecule is in the same lipoprotein subtype as other LDL particles, as it contains a single molecule of Apo B100 embedded in the outer surface layer. Like a particle of LDL, the Lp(a) particle consists of a hydrophilic outer layer composed of phospholipids and free cholesterol and a hydrophobic central core of triglycerides and cholesterol esters. It is distinguished from LDL, however, by having one additional apolipoprotein bound to its outer surface, called apo(a). The apo (a) apolipoprotein is different than the Apo A apolipoprotein found on the surface of the HDL particle. A unique feature of apo(a) is that it is very similar to plasminogen, an important protein involved in the process of blood clotting.

Lp(a) appears to be a multiheaded villain. It has the same potential for depositing cholesterol as does LDL, and has the additional feature of being able to promote blood clotting. Lp(a) is present in the arterial wall of plaque. It is known to bind to macrophages in a way that enhances LDL accumulation and the macrophages' development into foam cells. It has also been shown to have a role in promoting endothelial cell dysfunction by increasing the likelihood of LDL penetration through endothelial cells. Lp(a) is known to promote recruitment of inflammatory cells into the intima. It has also been shown to promote smooth muscle cell growth and their infiltration into the intima.

Lp(a)'s blood clotting capabilities arise from its close chemical and structural similarity to plasminogen, one of the protective proteins made by the body as an anti-clotting factor that works at the site of blood clots to help dissolve the clot. Since Lp(a) is similar to plasminogen, it competes for receptors for plasminogen on cells as well as on the newly forming blood clot itself. By competing for plasminogen receptors, Lp(a) reduces the effectiveness of naturally occurring plasminogen to dissolve blood clots. Lp(a) has been called the "heart attack protein," since it is so frequently found to be elevated in the blood of patients who experience a heart attack.

HDL. At least as important as cholesterol deposition, and maybe more so, is the process by which cholesterol is taken away from the artery.

This is the function of HDL, through the process of reverse cholesterol transport that we mentioned earlier. The HDL particle functions as the garbage truck for cholesterol to facilitate its removal and transport from the arterial wall back to the liver.

As we have discussed, HDL particles are uniquely distinguished from other lipoproteins by carrying the apolipoprotein Apo A on their surface. The Apo A apolipoprotein can be further subdivided into the more beneficial Apo A1 and the less beneficial Apo A2. It is the Apo A1 apolipoprotein that gives the HDL particle its signals to interact with cells to remove cholesterol, as well as the signals for the HDL particle to transport its cholesterol back to the liver.

HDLs, like LDLs, also have subtypes based upon their size and density. Newly formed HDL particles are typically disk shaped. While an HDL particle has the ability to extract cholesterol from cells, it becomes much more potent when acted upon by an enzyme in the bloodstream called lecithin-cholesterol acyl transferase, also known as LCAT. LCAT changes the smaller disk-shaped HDL to the larger, spherical HDL. The large, spherical HDL is more effective in the process of reverse cholesterol transport and appears to be the best variety of HDL for conferring protection against atherosclerosis. This spherical HDL is also known as HDL-2, or large, buoyant HDL by virtue of its size and density relative to other types of HDL.

If HDL is the garbage truck for the transport of cholesterol back to the liver, the subtypes of HDL can be considered as either full or empty garbage trucks. The poorly functioning disk-shaped HDLs are the lazy garbage trucks that circulate mostly empty of cholesterol. The large, spherical, HDL-2 are the hard working garbage trucks that circulate in the bloodstream mostly full and carrying garbage back to the dump (**figure 4.5**).

While higher HDL-C levels are correlated with cardiovascular health, no incremental increase in HDL has been proven to improve health. In other words, while high HDL-C levels might correlate with better cardiovascular health, specifically increasing one's HDL-C might not increase cardiovascular health or reduce the risk of CHD events and atherosclerosis.

The concept of the HDL particle as the "garbage truck" for cholesterol

Removal of Cholesterol by HDL From the Artery Back to the Liver

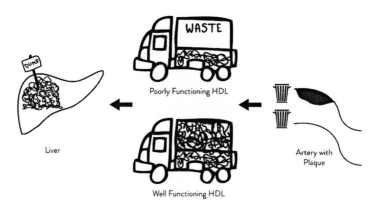

Figure 4.5 Legend: Removal of Cholesterol by HDL from the Artery Back to the Liver. When HDL is functioning well, it carries substantial amounts of cholesterol back to the liver, and can be thought of as a full garbage truck. When HDL is not functioning normally, there is a preponderance of empty garbage trucks.

Illumination: In many instances, low HDL levels correspond with a higher risk of CHD. In such cases, there are not enough garbage trucks taking the excess cholesterol back to the liver. However, sometimes a person may have a low level of HDL, but most of it is the most beneficial large HDL-2 variety. If this is the case, although there are fewer garbage trucks, those that are present are working very hard and are full of cholesterol. This may confer significant protection against atherosclerosis.

In a region of Italy, a cluster of related individuals has been identified who produce abnormal and apparently more efficient HDL. This has been called the Apo A1Milano variant. These individuals actually have low measured HDL-C levels yet very low rates of cardiovascular events, even with high blood cholesterol values. Conversely, sometimes there may be a normal or even high level of HDL, but most of it is the small, disk-shaped variety of HDL. In this case, there are plenty of garbage trucks around, but very few are actually hauling garbage.

Vascular Inflammation

Inflammation in the arterial wall is as critical a component of atherosclerosis as endothelial dysfunction and LDL cholesterol accumulation. The body's inflammatory response is what leads to the formation of foam cells, without which there would be no fatty streak and subsequent development of plaque. Inflammation is a normal and necessary bodily function. In the case of atherosclerosis, however, inflammation is maladaptive. It actually fuels the atherosclerotic process. Halting and reversing plaque growth requires not only reducing cholesterol buildup but also extinguishing inflammation.

We have already discussed the central role that white blood cells such as monocytes, lymphocytes and macrophages play in inflammation and how they serve to facilitate plaque development. A number of chemicals that are primarily released from these white blood cells also play central roles in initiating, maintaining and accelerating the inflammatory response. These include a group of chemicals called cytokines that are known by such names as interleukin-6, interleukin 18 and tumor necrosis factor-alpha (TNF-alpha). These substances remain an active area of scientific inquiry among medical researchers studying atherosclerosis.

The most dangerous forms of atherosclerotic plaque are those that display the most chronic inflammation. There are two chemicals that have been well studied and are noted to be intimately associated with the inflammatory response within plaque. One is called C-reactive protein (CRP). CRP is found not only in plaque, but is also measurable in the bloodstream. It is made by white blood cells and is considered an acute phase reactant, meaning that any inflammation in the body can cause the release of CRP. Thus, a sore throat, a twisted knee or a full-blown heart attack all cause CRP to be released. However, chronic elevations in small quantities of CRP, measured in the blood as hs-CRP (the hs standing for high sensitivity), are highly predictive of an increased risk of CHD.

Once thought to be an innocent bystander in atherosclerosis, CRP has now been shown to play a critical and varied role in the development of plaque as well as in the transition of plaque from stable plaque to vulnerable plaque. Among the roles found for CRP are facilitating the entry of LDL into macrophages, releasing cytokines involved in inflammation and inducing the expression of CAMs on endothelial cells.

A second chemical that may be even more important in the process of inflammation, and a more specific marker of inflammation in plaque, is known as lipoprotein-associated phospholipase A2 (Lp-PLA$_2$). Like CRP, it is made by white blood cells, but it can also be made in the liver. Unlike CRP, Lp-PLA$_2$ circulates in the bloodstream attached to lipoprotein particles, primarily LDL. It is believed to be delivered to the artery via the LDL particle. Once in the intimal layer of the artery, Lp-PLA$_2$ has several functions, one of which is promoting the oxidation of LDL. In the unique chemical process of LDL oxidation mediated by Lp-PLA$_2$, two additional chemicals are generated, called LysoPC and oxFA. Both of these chemicals are potent triggers of both inflammation and further plaque growth. Thus, Lp-PLA$_2$ may represent the "missing link" between LDL oxidation in the intimal layer of the artery and local inflammation in and around atherosclerotic plaque.

The Fate of Plaque

As we discussed in Chapter two, plaque can evolve into either stable plaque or vulnerable plaque. What influences plaque to go in one direction or the other is still uncertain. Stable plaque typically grows very slowly. It contains more calcium and less inflammation, which helps to make the plaque less prone to rupture. Recall that while stable plaque can cause gradual narrowing of the interior of the artery, it is not a frequent cause of a heart attack.

The more dangerous type of plaque is the vulnerable plaque. In coronary arteries, it is responsible for the majority of heart attacks. One distinguishing feature of vulnerable plaque is that the inflammatory response within it is much greater. Such plaque contains more monocytes, macrophages and lymphocytes. Vulnerable plaque also tends to have a thinner lining of endothelial cells (the fibrous capsule) overlying it. The processes of ongoing inflammation and plaque growth and a thin fibrous capsule set up the right environment for this type of plaque to rupture through the fibrous capsule.

When this occurs, the same CAMs on the endothelial cells that attracted inflammatory cells to the oxidized LDL become activated. A full-scale "intruder alert" is instituted, as the body mounts a potent anti-inflammatory response. The body also sends blood platelets to the region of rupture, which clump together and form a blood clot, as further described below. This is the most dangerous of all situations inside the blood vessel, because the combination of blood clot and cholesterol plaque leads to a sudden cutoff in blood supply.

We know from clinical and autopsy studies that plaque rupture occurs much more frequently than is recognized by the development of symptoms in the individual. In fact, the process of plaque rupture and occlusion of arteries may occur quite frequently, only to be aborted by the body's natural anti-clotting and healing mechanisms. However, if the environment for endothelial dysfunction, plaque growth and inflammation persists, the same area of plaque may continue to remain active. If the rupture is large enough, and the body's natural defenses are incapable of containing the rupture, the result may be catastrophic.

If this occurs in a major coronary artery, a large area of heart muscle can lose its oxygen supply. This can lead to permanent damage to the muscle and the development of scar tissue. However, the most dangerous consequence is that the abrupt interruption of oxygen to heart muscle can trigger erratic heart rhythms that can lead to a profound drop in blood pressure. This further deprives both the heart and brain of oxygen. Unless prompt treatment is administered, this scenario results in the syndrome of sudden cardiac death. Unfortunately, this is not a rare event, as it occurs over 300,000 times a year in the United States.

Arterial Thrombosis

The scenario described above is a sentinel example of the interaction among cholesterol, endothelial dysfunction, inflammation and clot formation. Clot formation is known as thrombosis, since the blood protein thrombin is involved in the crucial step of forming a blood clot. The development of blood clots plays an important role in many of the acute illnesses caused by atherosclerosis, such as stroke and myocardial infarction. Formation of blood clots generally is not a significant contributor to the growth of stable cholesterol plaque in the arterial wall. However, a number of changes occur in the diseased area of the artery where plaque is growing that enhance the potential for clot formation.

One such change is the endothelial dysfunction and the expression of CAMs on endothelial cells that makes these cells sticky, so they attract and hold onto platelets, the main clotting cell in the bloodstream. Platelets are a significant component of the disease processes of atherosclerosis leading to strokes and heart attacks. The inflammatory response that occurs inside the arterial wall also generates clotting factors in this region that can promote blood clot development under the right circumstances. These clotting factors include such substances as fibrinogen, plasminogen activator inhibitor-1, von Willebrand factor and D-dimer. Finally, particles such as Lp(a), when present in plaque and the bloodstream, serve to counteract the body's clot-dissolving mechanisms. Ultimately the result is the development of a blood clot in the artery that occludes the blood flow within the artery.

PART II

The Clinical Aspects of Atherosclerosis

Chapter 5

Cardiac Risk Factors:

Sugar and Spice (and Everything Else Not So Nice)

AS WE LEARNED in previous chapters, atherosclerosis is a complex process that involves endothelial dysfunction, cholesterol deposition, inflammation and sometimes thrombosis. We also learned that cholesterol deposition occurs through the entry of Apo B100-containing particles, primarily LDL, into the arterial wall. This requires an elevation of LDL-cholesterol (LDL-C) in the bloodstream, and while this is a necessary condition for atherosclerosis to occur, it is usually, in and of itself, not always a sufficient condition for atherogenesis. This is where additional cardiac risk factors play a significant role in determining whether atherosclerosis and the illnesses that develop as a result of atherosclerosis will occur.

In some cases the risk factor directly affects the likelihood of lipid deposition into the arterial wall by altering the composition of blood lipids. In some instances, the risk factor affects the other components of the atherosclerosis process: endothelial dysfunction, arterial inflammation or thrombosis. In many instances, more than one part of the atherosclerosis process is affected.

Some of these risk factors are modifiable, meaning they can be altered to either reduce or increase one's risk of developing atherosclerosis. Some risk factors are non-modifiable, meaning they cannot be altered. Examples of non-modifiable risk factors include age, gender and family history. Even though one may have non-modifiable risk factors, proper treatment of coexisting risk factors can still substantially reduce cardiovascular risk.

This chapter will provide an overview of the many medical conditions that represent cardiovascular risk factors. The more risk factors you have, the greater the risk of atherosclerosis. In fact, as the number of major risk factors increases, the risk of atherosclerosis does not increase geometrically, but rather increases exponentially. What this means is that if you have two major risk factors, your risk of atherosclerosis is twice as high as if you had one risk factor. However, if you have three major risk factors, your risk is not three times higher but instead is nine times higher than if you had just one risk factor. By recognizing that cardiovascular risk is exponentially associated with the number of risk factors, it should be clear that reducing or eliminating even one major risk factor can substantially reduce your risk of coronary heart disease (CHD).

There are many modifiable risk factors for CHD. Among the major ones are diabetes, cigarette smoking, high blood pressure, being overweight or obese, physical inactivity and abnormalities in blood lipids. There are numerous other, non-major risk factors. We do not term them "minor" risk factors, since they are also clearly associated with an increased risk of CHD. However, these risk factors are frequently cofactors or occur in association with other major risk factors. Thus, it is very difficult to exactly determine their precise influence on the development of CHD. In some cases, the non-major risk factors may contribute significantly to the likelihood of an individual developing CHD or experiencing an MI (myocardial infarction) or a CVA (cerebrovascular accident or stroke).

Some of the common non-major risk factors, to name only a few, include: (1) an unhealthy diet that is low in fruits and vegetables and high in saturated fats, (2) chronic and excessive stress, (3) chronic kidney problems, (4) heavy alcohol use, (5) use of certain medications, such as hormone supplements, (6) low socioeconomic status, (7) mental illness and (8) an inflammatory state in which there are elevated levels of Lp(a) and CRP in the bloodstream. As there are nearly 400 cardiac risk factors, the discussion below covers many of the most common, but certainly not all of the important CHD risk factors.

Unhealthy Diet

Dietary therapy remains the first step in the treatment of lipid abnormalities. Unhealthy diets promote many lipid abnormalities that contribute to CHD including an elevation in Total Cholesterol and LDL-C, an increase in triglycerides, unfavorable changes in the ratio of good and bad cholesterol, increased levels of other atherogenic particles such as VLDL, IDL, small, dense LDL, Apo B100, Lp(a) and the number of LDL particles.

Before we can discuss what a heart-healthy diet is, we need to establish what foods have unhealthy effects. Unhealthy foods that promote clogging of the arteries are: (1) those high in saturated fats, trans-fats and dietary cholesterol, (2) those high in sodium, because they increase risk of hypertension, and (3) those high in refined sugar and starches, because they increase the risk of diabetes and metabolic syndrome.

We previously reviewed the findings of the Seven Countries Study, which established for the first time the link between consumption of saturated fat and risk of developing CHD and stroke. Ongoing analysis of data from this same study found that after 25 years of follow-up, the risk of dying from CHD due to saturated fat consumption was also much higher. Furthermore, the risk of dying from CHD was also associated with an increased consumption of dietary cholesterol and trans-fats.

What are dietary fats and cholesterol? All fats are composed of molecules of triglyceride. Triglycerides are made up of a chemical backbone of one molecule glycerol and three fatty acid chains (hence the name tri-glyceride). There are three varieties of fatty acids, classified according to how "saturated" they are. Saturation is the chemical term that reflects the number of hydrogen atoms attached to the carbon atoms in the fatty acid. More hydrogen atoms make the fatty acid chain shorter and denser. Because saturated fats are denser, they are typically solid at room temperature.

Saturated Fats. Unlike cholesterol, which is found only in animal-derived products, saturated fats are found in both animal and plant products. Typical examples of foods high in saturated fats would be butter, fat associated with meat, lard, full-fat dairy products like whole milk and cheese, fried foods and tropical oils like coconut and palm-kernel oil. The recommended level of saturated fat intake is to consume less than seven percent of total daily calories from saturated fat. So for a typical 2,000-calorie diet, the saturated fat allowance is only 15 grams.

Alert! A McDonald's Quarter Pounder with cheese, two tablespoons of butter and a T-bone steak each contain 15 grams of saturated fat.

Saturated fats are more easily incorporated into the LDL particle. They also slow the activity of the LDL receptors on the liver, which are responsible for removing LDL particles from the bloodstream. As a result of this, saturated fats are more likely to raise LDL-C. They also impair endothelial function and increase arterial inflammation, thus promoting LDL oxidation. Saturated fats also inhibit the protective effects of HDL. Finally, saturated fats increase insulin secretion, which can lead to insulin resistance, a subject we will discuss in more detail in the sections on diabetes and metabolic syndrome.

The healthier triglycerides are the monounsaturated and polyunsaturated fats, which have fewer hydrogen molecules in their fatty acid chains. These fats are liquid at room temperature, and are therefore known as oils. Examples of monounsaturated fats would be the fat in olive oil, avocados and most nuts. The most common examples of polyunsaturated fats are the omega-3 oils that come from marine life. Monounsaturated and polyunsaturated fats are much more heart-healthy than saturated fats and are a major component of the heart-healthy diets we will discuss later.

Excessive caloric intake, alcohol and high carbohydrate diets also contribute to the elevation of blood triglycerides. Even without weight loss, reducing calories and alcohol intake will improve blood lipids. Very low fat, high carbohydrate diets like the Pritikin and Ornish diets may paradoxically increase triglyceride and LDL levels, especially in patients who have insulin resistance associated with diabetes or metabolic syndrome.

Trans-Fats. Another source of bad fat is trans-fat. Trans-fats are not natural fats, but instead are created when manufacturers turn liquid polyunsaturated vegetable oil into a solid fat by chemically adding hydrogen, a process known as hydrogenation. This process modifies inexpensive vegetable oil to make the fat more stable, and so preserve shelf life, texture and taste of many commonly consumed products. Many brands of margarine and shortening contain trans-fats, and so do many fried and baked products that are cooked with these fats. However, because they are so prevalent in commercial foods and foods we buy at the supermarket, trans-fats are a major public health hazard, just as cigarettes are.

Like other saturated fats, trans-fats also increase LDL-C. They also change the shape of LDL particles into the more dangerous small, dense particles that more easily cross the endothelium to form the core of arterial plaque. Trans-fats also increase inflammation in the artery, raise triglycerides, lower HDL-C and raise Lp(a) (the heart attack protein). It is therefore no surprise that trans-fats are even more dangerous than saturated fats with respect to increasing the risk of CHD.

In the Nurses' Health Study of 84,000 women, those consuming the highest levels of trans-fat had a 67 percent higher risk of CHD events over eight years of follow-up, when compared to those consuming the lowest levels of trans-fat. Another study looking at the relationship between the amount of trans-fat and CHD risk found that just a two percent increase in dietary trans-fat intake was associated with an astounding 23 percent increase in CHD.

As of 2006, the U.S. government has required food manufacturers to list trans-fat on the 'Nutrition Facts' panel of commercial foods. Although it is recommended that you consume zero grams of trans-fat, a product that contains less than 0.5 gram of trans-fat per serving can still call itself trans-fat free. If the words *hydrogenated*, *partially hydrogenated* or *shortening* are listed on the 'Nutrition Facts' panel of a product, the product contains trans-fat. Keep in mind that restaurants, bakers and bulk food producers are not required to report trans-fat content. Remarkably, the food served in many hospital and school cafeterias has been found to be loaded with trans-fats.

Alert! A hospital cafeteria may be one of the least healthy places to eat. Study after study has shown that hospital cafeterias prepare food with higher trans-fat, saturated fat, cholesterol and sodium content than most restaurants. Soft drink machines and "impulse" snacks line the hallways and cashier aisles of many hospital cafeterias. Worst of all, a recent survey found that 89 percent of U.S. hospitals and 50 percent of Canadian hospitals had fast-food outlets on site. So, not only can you get the Burger King food while you visit or work at the hospital, but you get it at the hospital discount price!

Public awareness has significantly reduced trans-fat consumption. Since 2005, the amount of trans-fat being put in our food has declined by 50 percent. Many communities such as New York City have banned trans-fat use in restaurants.

Alert! Public health campaigns have been successful in reducing the trans-fat content of many commercial goods. However, some fast-food brands of french fries still contain up to ten grams of trans-fat, doughnuts up to five grams, and many commercially baked cookies contain two and a half grams of trans-fat per serving.

Cholesterol. Dietary cholesterol is not a fat. It is a molecule made only by animals. We have already reviewed the chemistry and biology of cholesterol and learned that it is vital for life. However, all of the cholesterol our body needs can be manufactured by our liver. Therefore, any ingested cholesterol is, in effect, unnecessary. Diets high in cholesterol raise LDL levels in two ways. One is to make more cholesterol directly available to the LDL particle. The second is to impair removal of cholesterol by depressing the activity of the liver's LDL receptors.

Cholesterol is found in meat, chicken, fish, milk products and eggs. Organ meats (like liver pâté), egg yolks, poultry skin and marbleized red meats are especially high in cholesterol. The recommended amount of daily cholesterol intake is no more than 200 milligrams. Thus, being careful when eating meat, eggs and dairy products will help to keep you within your cholesterol intake guidelines.

> **Alert!** Liver pâté has 500 milligrams of cholesterol per serving. A single egg contains 150–220 milligrams of cholesterol, almost all of it in the yolk.

Obesity

Most of us think of obesity as simply a state of being overweight. However, obesity is a medical condition in which excess body fat has accumulated to an extent that it may have adverse effects on health. Obesity increases the likelihood of various diseases, particularly heart disease, diabetes, obstructive sleep apnea, arthritis and certain types of cancer. It is most commonly caused simply by an imbalance in caloric intake and caloric expenditure. The consumption of excessive food energy combined with the lack of physical activity is responsible for 99 percent of obesity cases. There may be some genetic susceptibility, but hormonal imbalances, medications and psychiatric illnesses only rarely cause obesity.

Obesity is viewed as one of the most serious public health problems of the 21st century. The incidence and prevalence of overweight and obesity have increased dramatically in the United States in the last generation. In 1960, about 15 percent of women and 10 percent of men were classified as obese. In 2000, these numbers had risen so much that 65 percent of all adults were classified as either overweight or obese, with 35 percent of women and 25 percent of men meeting the definition of obesity. Perhaps of even greater concern is the alarming rise in childhood obesity. Because childhood obesity often persists into adulthood and is associated with numerous chronic illnesses, children who are obese need to have early surveillance for hypertension, diabetes, cholesterol disorders and even CHD.

Obesity Measurement. Even though obesity is a state of being overweight, from a medical standpoint obesity is more specifically classified by the body mass index (BMI). Body mass index is defined as the individual's body weight divided by the square of his or her height. Although it has several limitations that we will discuss later, BMI is commonly used to provide a simple numeric measure of a given individual's "fatness" or "thinness." Charts and online calculators for BMI are readily available.

> **Illumination:** You can quickly determine your BMI by knowing your height and weight. BMI is expressed in metric units of kg/m². By using the following simple formula, entering weight in pounds and height in inches will allow you to calculate your BMI in metric units:
>
> BMI = [weight (in pounds) x 703] / [height (in inches)]²
>
> Thus, for a typical individual weighing 170 pounds and 5'10" (70 inches) tall:
>
> BMI = [170 x 703] / [70]² = 23 kg/m²

Typically a BMI between 18.5 and 25 kg/m² is considered ideal. A person with a BMI above 25 kg/m² meets the definition of being overweight, while one above 30 kg/m² is considered obese. A BMI above 40 kg/m² classifies a person as morbidly obese. In Asian populations these standards are lower.

While BMI is a well-accepted measure of obesity, it has several flaws. It does not take into account muscle mass. Thus, some patients with an elevated BMI may actually be quite lean, because they have a large amount of muscle contributing to lean body mass and have a low percentage of body fat. BMI provides no information about weight distribution; that is, where your fat resides. Those individuals with the healthier "pear" shape may have the same BMI as those with the less healthy "apple" shape. Finally, because BMI requires the taking of two measurements (height and weight) and the use of a mathematical formula, it can be complex to calculate and track over time.

Other obesity measures seek to overcome some of these limitations. Waist circumference has been found to be closely associated with BMI and is much easier to measure, since neither height nor weight need be measured. To measure waist circumference, start by locating your hip bone and snugly (without compressing the skin) wrap a tape measure around your bare waist at this level. Make sure you are not holding your breath, and that the tape measure remains horizontal and at an even level all the way around your waist.

> **Illumination:** We traditionally think of the waist to be at the level of the belly button. In reality, the waist circumference measurement used in the definition of obesity is actually a hip circumference measurement.

For Caucasians and blacks, a normal waist circumference is less than 35 inches for women and less than 40 inches for men. For Asians, as with BMI, the waist circumference thresholds are lower. Waist circumference specifically measures central obesity or belly fat. Central obesity, characterized by the "apple-shaped" body type, features the kind of fat deposition that is most closely associated with CHD risk. It is also the type of obesity that most commonly promotes the development of metabolic syndrome and diabetes, both of which are major CHD risk factors.

An index that offers some advantages over both BMI and waist circumference is the waist:hip ratio. It is calculated by measuring the waist circumference at the level of the belly button, and the hip circumference at the widest point of the hips, typically at the level of the buttocks. While not specifically an obesity measure, it provides more information about the distribution of fat. Since abdominal fat, also termed visceral fat, is the unhealthiest (and in excess becomes the condition of central obesity), having a way to estimate abdominal fat relative to other areas of fat distribution is of value. A waist:hip ratio of greater than 1.0 indicates a large amount of belly or visceral fat and signifies patients at increased risk of CHD and metabolic problems due to obesity. A waist:hip ratio of less than 0.9 is considered in the fit range.

Not only is the incidence of diabetes and metabolic syndrome increased in obese and overweight patients, so are the other major CHD risk factors of hypertension and abnormal lipid levels. Central obesity in particular leads to an overproduction of VLDL lipoproteins by the liver, which in turn leads to a rise in LDL-C. For these reasons, the risk of CHD illnesses and death are significantly increased in centrally obese individuals.

> **Alert!** A BMI above 32 kg/m² is associated with a doubled mortality rate in women. On average, obesity reduces life expectancy by six to seven years. Morbid obesity, signified by a BMI over 40 kg/m², reduces life expectancy by ten years.

Since obesity is primarily caused by an accumulation and growth of fat cells caused by caloric intake that is in excess of expenditure, the primary treatment for obesity is to reduce both. Reducing the consumption of energy-dense foods, such as those high in fat, sugar and complex carbohydrates, and increasing dietary fiber intake are the mainstays in the dietary management of obesity. Equally important is a regular exercise regimen that emphasizes aerobic activity, which results in the burning of calories.

In most cases, diet and exercise regimens are effective, at least in the short term. The maintenance of weight loss is more problematic. Various psychological and social factors contribute to the high incidence of weight regain in overweight and obese patients. The long-term success rates of most weight-loss programs range from two percent to 20 percent. In patients with medical illnesses directly caused by their obesity, there is a role for anti-obesity medications as well as bariatric surgical procedures.

Diabetes

Diabetes mellitus, or simply diabetes, is a condition that results from the body's inability to produce and/or use insulin. Insulin is a hormone made by the pancreas that is necessary for the body to transport sugar circulating in the bloodstream into cells where it can be converted into cellular energy. The lack of insulin, or response to insulin, causes most diabetics to have elevated blood sugar.

There are two types of diabetes. Type 1 diabetes is relatively uncommon. It is usually diagnosed in children and young adults. In type 1 diabetes, the pancreas makes no insulin, thus making it necessary for all type I diabetics to be treated with periodic insulin injections or by an insulin pump.

Type 2 diabetes is the most common form of diabetes, accounting for 95 percent of all cases of diabetes. In type 2 diabetes either the body does not produce enough insulin or, more commonly, the cells do not respond to insulin, a condition known as insulin resistance, abbreviated as IR. This lack of response causes the body to make even more insulin. Thus, unlike the type 1 diabetic, whose insulin levels are low, the type 2 diabetic with insulin resistance actually has high insulin levels. However, the insulin is not effective because the cells of the body have stopped responding to insulin.

The signs and symptoms of diabetes are extremely variable. The typical symptoms include frequent urination, excessive thirst, fatigue and the seeming paradox of extreme hunger accompanied by weight loss. In fact, diabetes was at one time described as "starvation in the midst of plenty." Numbness and tingling in the feet and legs, blurred vision and slow-healing bruises and cuts may also occur. Testing for diabetes is quite easy, requiring only a fasting blood sample to measure glucose. This is the main form of sugar in the body, and a fasting level above 100–110 mg/dL is considered suggestive of diabetes.

There are currently 25 million type 2 diabetics in the United States, or about eight percent of the population. An additional 50 million adults have impaired glucose tolerance, also known as prediabetes. Particularly alarming is the trend showing that an additional two million Americans are developing diabetes every year.

Insulin Resistance. While insulin resistance (IR) is an essential component of type 2 diabetes, the syndrome of IR also occurs in patients without diabetes. It is also a feature of other cardiac risk factors discussed in this chapter, such as metabolic syndrome, obesity and hypertension. IR has both genetic and environmental determinants. In most instances though, a genetic predisposition is unmasked by environmental factors, such as obesity, a sedentary lifestyle and cigarette smoking, which result in the development of IR. Obesity is the strongest risk factor for the development of IR and diabetes.

To understand insulin resistance, it is necessary to appreciate the functions of insulin. Insulin has been called the "master metabolic hormone." It is made primarily in the pancreas, which sits next to the liver and behind the stomach in the abdomen. Its primary function is to allow glucose to enter cells, where it can be utilized in the generation of cellular energy. Glucose is the main form in which sugars circulate in our bloodstream. However, insulin has a number of other important functions related to the regulation of both sugar and fat metabolism. These include: (1) controlling the production of glucose and the metabolism of carbohydrates by the liver, (2) suppression of the release of fatty acids from fat tissue into the circulation, and (3) promoting the breakdown of circulating triglycerides into their component fat particles and the subsequent uptake of these particles into cells. When IR develops, all of these functions may be impaired to varying degrees.

In its early stages, IR may not result in elevated levels of blood glucose, as the body is able to compensate by making more insulin. As IR progresses to diabetes, blood glucose levels become elevated. The atherosclerosis that develops in patients with IR and diabetes is due not to elevated blood sugar levels but rather to the loss of some of the normal lipid-regulating effects of insulin.

IR and obesity are closely linked. In most cases, obesity results not from an increase in the number of fat cells, but rather from an increase in the size of fat cells. The increased size of fat cells promotes the release of fatty acids normally contained inside fat cells into the circulation. Fatty acids in the bloodstream impair the lipid-regulating effects of insulin. Abdominal fat, also known as visceral fat, is the most metabolically active type of fat, and so contributes disproportionally to the levels of circulating fatty acids. This is the reason belly fat is so much worse metabolically than fat accumulation anywhere else in the body.

The primary lipid metabolic abnormality in IR is an overproduction by the liver of VLDL particles, which is induced by a high level of circulating fatty acids. An excessive production of VLDL particles leads to three lipid abnormalities, all of which promote the development of atherosclerosis; elevated triglycerides, reduced HDL-C and a predominance of small, dense LDL particles. This constellation of abnormalities is termed *atherogenic dyslipidemia*. As we know from the sections on plaque development, all of these abnormalities significantly contribute to the formation of atherosclerotic plaque.

Diabetes is considered a CHD risk equivalent. What this means is that, more than being a CHD risk factor, just having diabetes is considered equivalent to a diagnosis of CHD. Between 50 percent and 70 percent of all deaths in diabetics are due to CHD. The risk of CHD, stroke and peripheral vascular disease (PVD) is two to four times higher in diabetics than nondiabetics. This also means that diabetics should be treated with the same level of aggressiveness as a patient who already has a diagnosis of CHD.

The management of IR, diabetes and the resultant metabolic abnormalities requires a two-fold approach. Lifestyle changes are the first step. These require both increased physical activity and weight reduction. Both improve insulin sensitivity. Controlling cigarette smoking and excessive alcohol intake is vital, as both contribute to IR. The second step is to use medications to both control lipids and reverse IR. We will discuss both of these approaches further in subsequent chapters.

Metabolic Syndrome

IR plays a central role in the development of a cluster of interrelated metabolic abnormalities called metabolic syndrome. This is also known as the cardiometabolic risk syndrome, because of the frequent association of CHD with these metabolic abnormalities. This syndrome was at one time considered to be prediabetes and is certainly a risk factor for the development of diabetes later in life. Metabolic syndrome in and of itself is also a major risk factor for CHD.

Components. There are five core components of metabolic syndrome: (1) obesity, (2) atherogenic dyslipidemia, (3) elevated blood pressure, (4) elevated blood glucose and (5) elevated markers in the bloodstream of inflammation and enhanced blood clotting. Of these five components, obesity is believed to be the primary modulator and cause of metabolic syndrome. In almost all individuals with metabolic syndrome, central or visceral obesity is present. Obesity can be defined by either the BMI or waist circumference thresholds. The metabolically active belly fat releases high amounts of fatty acids into the circulation, which are primarily responsible for the development of IR. Belly fat may also contribute to an enhanced state of inflammation in the bloodstream, which is also believed to play a role in the disease processes associated with metabolic syndrome.

The atherogenic dyslipidemia associated with metabolic syndrome is the same as that discussed in the section on IR and diabetes, causing abnormalities that include elevated triglycerides (>150 mg/dL), reduced HDL-C (<40 mg/dL) and a predominance of small, dense LDL particles. Elevated blood pressure (BP) is defined by either a BP of 130/85 mmHg or greater or the patient's use of blood pressure medications to control BP. Elevated blood glucose is defined as a fasting level greater than 100–110 mg/dL or the use of diabetic medications.

Markers of inflammation and enhanced blood clotting (thrombosis) are frequently present in metabolic syndrome. Similar to the association of obesity with IR, central obesity appears to also directly cause the enhanced inflammatory and clotting responses seen in metabolic syndrome. An elevated CRP level is the most commonly recognized inflammatory marker. Other markers of arterial inflammation are also present. These can arise from two sources: signs that indicate endothelial cells have been triggered to display their inflammatory surface receptors, and signs that indicate inflammation is occurring below the endothelium as a result of increased oxidation of the LDL particle.

An increase in thrombosis is caused by the stickiness of blood platelets and contributes to the increased risk of blood clotting in metabolic syndrome. This is reflected in the increased likelihood of both stroke and MI, both of which are associated with blood clotting caused by sticky platelets in the artery. One link between atherosclerosis and thrombosis we have already discussed is the Lp(a) particle that is found in association with LDL. Many patients with both diabetes and metabolic syndrome have elevated levels of Lp(a).

Alert! Like diabetes, the prevalence of metabolic syndrome is high and rising. Metabolic syndrome affects almost 50 percent of the U.S. population over the age of 50. More women than men have metabolic syndrome. Half of all patients with CHD have metabolic syndrome, and it is present in over one-third of patients with CHD before the age of 45.

Treatments aimed at metabolic syndrome are usually directed against its individual components. Thus, weight loss, control of lipids, blood pressure and blood sugar, and antiplatelet agents like aspirin are mainstays of therapy. The search for a single defect in metabolism caused by central obesity has been ongoing, but its discovery remains elusive. Until such a discovery is made, many experts believe that treatment of IR through drugs used to treat diabetes should be a cornerstone of therapy in patients with metabolic syndrome.

High Blood Pressure

Hypertension or high blood pressure is as important a risk factor for CHD as are lipid abnormalities. With respect to the risk of stroke and CVD, hypertension may be an even more important risk factor than lipid abnormalities. Measuring blood pressure simply requires a cuff that wraps around the arm and measures the level of pressure generated by the beating heart as it is transmitted into the arteries of the body. While many of the current BP measuring devices are digital and/or electronic, BP was initially measured in the same way as barometric pressure in the atmosphere, with a mercury manometer. Therefore, BP readings are expressed according to the level that would be reached in a column of mercury, expressed as "mmHg" (Hg being the chemical symbol of mercury).

A BP result consists of two numbers. The higher reading is termed the *systolic blood pressure*; it reflects the pressure generated each time the heart squeezes to push blood forward, the phase of the cardiac cycle known as systole. The lower reading is the *diastolic pressure*, the pressure that remains in the arteries during diastole, the second phase of the cardiac cycle, when the heart is relaxed. Normal blood pressure is defined as a systolic blood pressure of less than 120 mmHg and/or a diastolic blood pressure of less than 80 mmHg.

Like lipid disorders, hypertension also affects 100 million Americans. The risk of developing hypertension has been steadily increasing, and currently there is a 90 percent chance that an individual in the United States will develop hypertension. Thus, it is a major risk factor. Hypertension causes arteriosclerosis, also known as hardening of the arteries. This process results in endothelial dysfunction, inflammation and an increased risk of thrombosis, just as atherosclerosis does.

> **Alert!** Like people with lipid disorders, the majority of patients with hypertension have no symptoms. Only 70 percent of individuals with hypertension are aware they have it. And even among those receiving medical care, BP is controlled in only 30 percent of individuals.

Inflammation. Many researchers believe that inflammation is the main disorder that occurs at the level of the artery in hypertension. Markers of vascular inflammation like CRP and lipoprotein-associated phospholipase A2 (Lp-PLA2) are frequently elevated in advanced stages of hypertension. Hypertension also promotes growth of the smooth muscle cells in the medial layer of the artery. This growth may cause an imbalance in the oxygen supply and demand for the arterial wall and so promote further endothelial dysfunction, inflammation and stress on the arterial wall. These abnormalities then make it easier for cholesterol accumulation in the artery. In this way, the arteriosclerosis that accompanies hypertension also promotes the development of atherosclerosis.

An ideal BP at all ages is believed to be no greater than 120/80 mmHg. When BP levels exceed these values, initial treatment involves lifestyle modifications. Many of the same lifestyle modifications used to treat lipid disorders are also used to lower BP, including weight reduction, aerobic exercise, smoking cessation and stress management. In addition to a lowered fat and sugar intake, lowering salt intake to less than 1,500 milligrams of sodium per day is vital. This can be accomplished through the DASH diet (Dietary Approach to Stop Hypertension), which especially emphasizes fruits, vegetables and low-fat or fat-free dairy products. Additionally, increasing dietary potassium, which offsets the effects of sodium, has been shown to be very effective in reducing BP. Dietary sources of potassium include bananas, citrus fruits, most vegetables and salt substitutes. Discontinuing tobacco use and limiting alcohol intake to less than two standard drinks per day has also been shown to effectively lower BP.

If these measures do not adequately achieve ideal BP, there is substantial evidence that using medications to lower BP will prevent, treat and reverse atherosclerosis. There are a number of medications that work in a variety of ways available to lower BP. In almost all patients, a medication regimen that works and is well tolerated is possible, although it may require some trial and error to find the right regimen. For patients with existing CHD or lipid abnormalities, the only medications that are generally to be avoided are diuretics, also known as water pills, since these often worsen the lipid blood levels and may also promote dangerous heart arrhythmias through the depletion of blood minerals like potassium and magnesium.

Cigarette Smoking

Smoking harms nearly every organ in the body. Smoking is a major risk factor for all forms of atherosclerosis, including CHD, stroke, peripheral arterial disease and aortic aneurysms. Smoking can also promote acute cardiovascular illnesses such as MI, unstable angina, stroke and sudden death. Despite the decline in smoking rates in the general population in the last decade, rates of smoking are rising among teenagers and young adults. It is currently estimated that 23 percent of all high school students smoke.

In the United States it is estimated that about six million years of potential lives are lost each year due to smoking. At the age of 50 years, a smoker's risk of dying is three times higher than that of a nonsmoker. Researchers from the University of Bristol in England have determined that a smoker's lifespan is shortened by 11 minutes with each cigarette smoked.

> **Illumination:** The study from the University of Bristol used data compiled from 34,000 physicians over a 40 year period. The determination that the 11 minutes of life were lost for each cigarette consumed was as follows:
>
> 1. The difference in the average life expectancy between smokers and nonsmokers was six and a half years, equal to 3,416,400 minutes.
> 2. An adult smoking an average of 5,772 cigarettes (less than one pack per day) per year from age 17 until death at age 61 would consume an average total of 311,688 cigarettes.
> 3. Therefore 3,416,400 minutes/311,688 cigarettes = 11 minutes/cigarette.

Any amount of smoking is harmful, including second-hand or passive smoking. At the age of 50 years, one-half of all smokers have evidence of CHD when measured by coronary artery calcium scores, compared to only 35 percent of nonsmokers. Active smoking increases the likelihood of CHD by 80 percent, compared to the likelihood in nonsmokers. Passive smoking increases the risk by 30 percent. Smoking combined with other major risk factors, such as diabetes, is especially harmful. In women, smoking combined with use of oral contraceptives and estrogen replacement is also especially hazardous.

Mechanisms of Harm. There are a number of mechanisms by which smoking promotes atherosclerosis and the acute illnesses that result from atherosclerosis. One mechanism is impairment in endothelial function, which we know results in increased permeability of the endothelium to LDL particles. In addition, the normal endothelial function of vasoreactivity, which permits blood vessels to constrict and enlarge in response to various stimuli, is also impaired by smoking. In some cases, smoking will cause the endothelium to constrict so severely in the coronary arteries that a condition known as coronary vasospasm occurs. This can cause a severe and prolonged deprivation in blood to the heart and result in an MI or sudden death. This is analogous to an asthmatic developing spasm in the bronchial tubes that causes a reduction in airflow into the lungs.

A second mechanism by which smoking causes atherosclerosis is that it promotes inflammation in the blood vessels. Smokers have higher levels of pro-inflammatory molecules on their endothelial surfaces and thus attract white blood cells to the arterial wall. Smoking also makes LDL particles in the arterial wall more susceptible to oxidation. Thus, once the white blood cells penetrate the damaged endothelial wall, they can then act on the oxidized LDL particle to form plaque in a much more aggressive and rapid fashion.

Smoking also directly affects lipid particles. Smokers have higher levels of triglycerides and LDL-C. Smoking also depresses HDL, which in some cases can be very severe. With the increase in the availability of particles that deposit cholesterol in the arterial wall, and the reduction in the number and function of particles that remove cholesterol, atherosclerosis risk is increased.

Finally, two additional mechanisms are worth noting. The nicotine in tobacco smoke is a potent stimulant to the heart. It causes an increase in the pulse rate and blood pressure. It may be the mechanism by which smoking causes spasms of the coronary arteries. Smoking also affects the coagulant properties of blood, increasing a number of clotting factors to promote the development of blood clots. This is especially true in women who smoke and also use estrogens in the form of either oral contraceptives or hormonal replacement. It also affects the blood platelets, making them stickier, so that when they are attracted to an area of arterial damage, a blood clot will form more quickly and be larger than if the platelets were functioning normally.

Cessation of smoking is one of the most effective ways to lower an individual's cardiovascular risk. It is well known that a number of the adverse chemical and health effects of smoking reverse almost immediately after stopping. The heart risks associated with cigarette use also reverse quickly. Within one year of stopping smoking, a person's CHD risk drops to half of that of a smoker. In as little as five years, the risk of CHD and stroke is reduced to the same risk as nonsmokers. Beyond the personal health benefits of cigarette cessation, there are also significant public health benefits. In communities that have banned smoking in public places, it is possible to show, within only six months, a 60 percent drop in the risk of acute MI.

Genetic Factors

Your family history and genetic composition strongly influence your cardiovascular risk. At first glance this may seem inconsistent with this book's premise that you are in control of whether you develop CHD. In fact, for atherosclerosis and CHD, the interaction between genetics and environment has a tremendous influence, such that it is the very rare patient who will develop atherosclerosis purely on a genetic basis. Even in such patients early identification can allow treatment to begin before atherosclerosis is permitted to develop.

Familial Hypercholesterolemia. The most common inherited cause of high LDL levels is a condition known as familial hypercholesterolemia (FH). About 85 percent of cases are caused by a defect or deficiency of the liver LDL receptor that helps to remove LDL from the bloodstream. Chromosomal mutations of two specific genes, the APOB gene and the PCSK9 gene, both of which result in an overproduction of LDL and/or Apo B100, account for the other 15 percent of cases of FH. Two clues that suggest a diagnosis of FH are elevated levels of total cholesterol at a young age and a very strong family history of early heart disease.

There are two varieties of FH, homozygous and heterozygous. The more severe variety is homozygous, since it is caused by defects in both chromosomes inherited from each parent. Fortunately, this type is very rare, occurring in one in one million individuals. When present, homozygous FH causes cholesterol levels in excess of 500 mg/dL and always results in development of CHD and atherosclerosis in other arteries in the body at a very early age.

The heterozygous variety of FH, in which only one chromosome is dysfunctional, is fairly common. It occurs in one in 500 persons, or about 620,000 people in the United States and ten million patients worldwide. Certain ethnic groups have a predisposition to FH, including French Canadians,

Christian Lebanese, Ashkenazi Jews and South Africans of Dutch Afrikaner descent. In these populations the incidence can be as high as one in 100 individuals. LDL-C levels are typically 200–400 mg/dL, and these individuals also have much higher levels of Lp(a), the "heart attack protein."

> **Alert!** Familial hypercholesterolemia is four times more common than sickle-cell disease and five times more common than cystic fibrosis, yet most people have never heard of the disease.

Like most patients with abnormal blood lipids, patients with FH have few external signs or symptoms. The rare patient may show small lipid deposits under the skin, called xanthalesmas and xanthomas. Symptoms develop in later stages of FH, and are often life-threatening. Without treatment, 50 percent of men and 30 percent of women with FH develop CHD before the age of 60 years. The closest relatives (parents, siblings, and children) of patients with FH have a 50 percent chance of also having FH. Thus, early screening and treatment to lower cholesterol is now recommended for FH patients and their relatives, even in childhood (as early as two years of age), to reduce the risk of CHD.

Familial Combined Hyperlipidemia. Another commonly inherited condition is called familial combined hyperlipidemia (FCH). This is even more common than FH, occurring in one in 200 persons overall, and is present in one in five individuals in whom CHD develops before the age of 60. In FCH patients, the liver makes too many VLDL particles, causing elevations in triglycerides, LDL-C and total cholesterol, and a lower level of HDL-C. These patients are especially prone to CHD because they have more circulating LDL particles of the more dangerous small, dense variety. Like FH, early recognition and treatment of FCH can be lifesaving.

Medical researchers have identified a number of other inherited lipid disorders, affecting nearly all types of lipid particles and metabolic pathways. Genetic disorders that cause isolated abnormalities of HDL, triglycerides, lipid-controlling enzymes, receptors and other metabolic controls may make a significant contribution to CHD risk. However, in nearly all instances it is possible to modify lipid levels through lifestyle interventions and prescription therapy.

As all genetic disorders affecting cholesterol metabolism are silent and without any symptoms until the patient has an illness caused by atherosclerosis (MI, CVA, aneurysm, etc.), their identification requires a screening blood examination. For this reason, it is now recommended that all individuals have a blood lipid panel screening at the age of 20, and that children with a family history of premature CHD or high cholesterol or who have diabetes or are obese have a blood test between the ages of two and 18. There is, in fact, strong evidence to consider moving these screening guidelines to a younger age.

Kidney Disease

Long-standing and moderately severe kidney disease is a significant CHD risk factor. Since chronic kidney disease (CKD) affects between 10 percent and 15 percent of the U.S. population, this risk factor is also very prevalent. Patients with CKD are at much higher risk of CHD than those with normal kidney function, and the level of risk increases as the level of kidney function worsens. Those at the highest risk are patients whose CKD is so severe they need dialysis. In such patients there is a 20 times higher risk of death due to CHD.

The most common causes of CKD are hypertension and diabetes; both are major risk factors for CHD. Thus, patients with CKD are often predisposed to develop CHD based upon the same underlying illness that caused the CKD. However, CKD in and of itself causes a number of abnormalities that promote the development of atherosclerosis. Blood lipid levels in patients with CKD are a major contributor to atherosclerosis. Triglyceride levels are high, HDL-C levels are low, and the numbers of small-dense LDL particles are high. This is exactly the same atherogenic lipid abnormality in the IR patients we discussed in the sections on insulin resistance, diabetes, and metabolic syndrome. Additionally, CKD patients also have more endothelial dysfunction, inflammation and risk for thrombosis, essentially all of the abnormalities that facilitate the development of atherosclerosis as well as the acute illnesses of CHD and CVA.

CKD patients are considered to be in the highest risk category for CHD and often need very aggressive treatment of both their CKD and their lipid abnormalities to reduce the risk. These treatments involve aggressive counseling in lifestyle modifications as well as medications to drastically lower LDL-C levels.

Stress

Stress has long been recognized as a contributor to heart disease. The incidence of heart attack and sudden death has been shown to increase significantly following acute stresses such as hurricanes, earthquakes and tsunamis. Chronic stress also increases the likelihood of CHD. It is important to understand which types of stress promote the occurrence of heart disease and to take steps to minimize the influence of these stresses.

Not all stress is detrimental. Certain types of stress actually have benefits. Stress can be a motivator toward one's achievement of worthwhile goals and is an integral part of such pleasurable activities as athletic competition. It can be associated with exhilaration, joy and a sense of accomplishment. However, when stress makes people feel out of control, stimulating a perceived need to make difficult or undesirable changes in order to adapt to events and situations, deleterious psychological and physical responses may occur.

People can have adverse stress responses to highly significant situations, such as the natural disasters mentioned above, or to personal issues such as a death in the family or the loss of a job. However, most commonly, stress responses are to the ordinary hassles we all experience in our lives such as traffic jams, personal disagreements, deadlines or just a disruption of one's routine.

The body's response to stress is to release stress hormones such as cortisol, adrenaline and angiotensin. The latter two are the most potent known vasoconstrictors (substances that can cause arteries to squeeze down extremely hard). The release of these hormones helps to facilitate the body's adaptive "fight or flight" response. This response helps to maintain blood pressure so that maximal blood flow to vital organs is preserved. However, the stress hormone response can also be maladaptive, as it can cause sufficient stress on the wall of the artery to result in plaque rupture or severe spasm of the artery. Both of these conditions can result in reduced blood flow. As we have discussed, when this occurs, a heart attack or stroke can follow.

> **Alert!** Stress hormones exhibit natural fluctuations in their levels, called circadian rhythms. Most people have peaks in their stress hormones early in the morning, early in the workweek and in the cold winter months. This may account for the observation that more heart attacks and strokes occur between the hours of six and eleven a.m., on Mondays, and in the winter.

In many cases, stresses may be ongoing rather than sporadic. The ongoing and continuous exposure to stress causes release and maintenance of a high level of stress hormones. As these hormones persist, instead of being used up when the stress resolves, they can stimulate the heart to increase both heart rate and blood pressure on a chronic basis. This, in turn, causes tension on the arteries, in the same way as chronic exposure to elevated blood pressure does. This tension promotes endothelial dysfunction, arteriosclerosis and an increase in the tendency of platelets to become sticky and cause blood clots. The endothelial dysfunction in particular increases the susceptibility of the artery for deposition of LDL cholesterol.

Stress hormones also increase the likelihood of atherosclerosis in another way. The stress hormone cortisol promotes the mobilization of stores of fat within the body. This is generally a positive adaptation, since fat can be used for energy to assist in the body's physical response to stress. In the situation in which stress hormone levels are chronically elevated, however, the mobilized fat becomes available for incorporation into LDL particles, which in turn leads to atherosclerosis. This is the same situation that occurs in metabolic syndrome when fatty acids from stored central fat are released into the bloodstream. In fact, there is substantial evidence of a strong link between stress and metabolic syndrome.

Stress is closely linked to both depression and anxiety syndromes. Both of these conditions are associated with an increased risk of CHD events. Anxiety syndromes, in which there are rapid spikes in adrenaline, have been known to trigger heart attacks. One such commonly recognized syndrome is "broken heart syndrome," also known as takotsubo syndrome, which is especially common in women. A precipitating stressful event causes acute stress on the heart, causing the heart to enlarge and suddenly weaken. This can lead to arrhythmias, sudden death, CHF and permanent heart damage, all without any buildup of atherosclerotic plaque.

Depression is also commonly associated with CHD events and, when present, increases the risk of poorer outcomes. Thirty percent of all patients having an MI suffer from depression, and in those with the most severe depressive symptoms, there is a four-fold higher risk of death. Similar observations have been made in patients having heart surgery.

Type A Behavior. The clinical data on the adverse cardiovascular effects of both acute and chronic stress is overwhelming. As early as 1950, research showed that the number of stressful events in an individual's life correlated closely with the likelihood of a major illness such as a heart attack. This finding led to the work of two California cardiologists, Dr. Meyer Friedman and Dr. Ray Rosenman, who recognized that not all of their heart patients had high cholesterol or high fat diets, but that many exhibited specific types of stress behaviors.

Using their observations, they categorized these behavior patterns into the now familiar Type A and B categories. Type A behavior is characterized by a continuous, deeply ingrained struggle to overcome real and imaginary obstacles imposed by events, other people and especially time. Type A individuals are frequently impatient, easily irritated, suspicious and hostile. While more common in men, Type A behaviors can also occur in women, who generally share the same characteristics as men, with the exception of being less hostile. Type B behavioral responses to stress lack those features noted above that characterize Type A individuals.

In the Western Collaborative Group Study, which looked at 3,500 healthy men with Type A behavior in the 1960s, researchers found that

Type A was an independent risk factor for CHD. Men with Type A were twice as likely to develop CHD as Type B men. Furthermore, in patients who had already had a heart attack, Type A behavior significantly increased the likelihood of a second heart attack. These findings have been confirmed by the Framingham Heart Study. The Framingham trial has gone on to show that women with Type A behavior are four times more likely to get CHD than women who are Type B.

Even individuals subjected to adverse stresses who are not necessarily Type A have an increased risk of CHD. The INTERHEART study of 28,000 patients from 52 countries showed that patients who admitted that they felt "irritable, anxious, or had sleeping difficulties as a result of conditions at work or at home" had a more than twofold higher risk of having an MI. The MRFIT trial showed that chronic work stress and marital dissolution increased the risk of dying due to CHD by threefold. In the Caregiver Health Effects study of 800 subjects, caregivers who had the responsibility of taking care of a spouse with dementia were shown, over a four-year period, to have a 63 percent higher mortality than matched control subjects. Most recently, the Women's Health Study showed that women with high job-related stress were twice as likely to have an MI and 43 percent more likely to need heart surgery than women with lower job-related stress.

There is considerable evidence that our behavioral response to stress may be at least partially genetically mediated. Children as young as three years of age have been shown to have Type A profiles. Studies have shown that the identification of Type A behavior in college-age students predicted an increased risk of CHD later in life. Since we have already shown that CHD often begins early in childhood, these findings are not surprising.

The fact that genetics may play a role in behavioral patterns that increase the risk of CHD does not necessarily mean that changing these patterns will not have a favorable outcome. Regular aerobic exercise reduces the level of circulating stress hormones. It is likely that exercise on a regular basis helps to "burn off" the hormonal elevations that occur in exposure to chronic stress. Likewise, counseling, psychotherapy, relaxation techniques, biofeedback and other anxiety- and anger-management techniques and forms of behavior modification can be useful in helping people relieve stress. There is ample evidence that patients with CHD who receive stress-management services have a reduced the risk of future CHD events and complications. In one study from San Francisco, the Recurrent Coronary Prevention Program, patients with CHD who lessened their Type A behavior had a 50 percent reduced risk of recurrent heart attacks after four years of follow-up than a control group that received no behavioral-modification training.

Cardiovascular responses to stress, like many of the body's responses, are adaptive to a point. When they become maladaptive, because of very high levels of stress, prolonged exposure to stress, or various behavioral and genetic predispositions, they have adverse effects on the heart. However, like other cardiovascular risk factors, stress risk can also be modified. This requires recognizing and understanding the risk and taking the appropriate actions to intervene. While it cannot be conclusively stated that stress causes CHD, stress can certainly aggravate CHD and result in poorer outcomes.

Inflammatory and Infectious Diseases

Recent evidence indicates that there is a link between certain illnesses that are characterized by an increase in the body's inflammatory state and CHD. This is not at all surprising given the key role that inflammation plays in the development of both stable and unstable atherosclerotic plaque. A number of systemic inflammatory diseases are associated with CHD. These include rheumatoid arthritis, psoriasis, inflammatory bowel disease and lupus.

Rheumatoid Arthritis. One of the best-studied links is between rheumatoid arthritis (RA) and CHD. RA is a chronic autoimmune disease that causes pain, swelling, stiffness and loss of function in multiple joints. It is characterized by both localized inflammation in joint spaces and an inflammatory response throughout the body. As it affects over two million Americans, most of whom are women between the ages of 20 and 50 years, RA is an especially prevalent, serious and often debilitating illness that strikes individuals in the prime of their life.

A Mayo Clinic study of more than 1,200 patients followed for over 40 years found that patients with RA were at a threefold higher risk of MI and a twofold higher risk of sudden death due to CHD than age-matched subjects without RA. Since the perception of pain is often altered in RA patients because they chronically take painkillers, this study also found that there was a fivefold higher risk of silent MIs in RA patients.

It also does not appear to take years for the development of CHD in patients with RA. A recent Swedish study found that the risk of an MI in patients with RA increases by 60 percent within the first year of diagnosis. Especially in women with RA, the risk of CHD is doubled. The use of pain-relieving therapies in RA, including NSAID medications, steroids and the newer COX-2 inhibitors like celecoxib (Celebrex), can also increase the risk of CHD as well as delay the detection of CHD symptoms. Since most patients with RA and CHD also have other CHD risk factors, early treatment to both modify traditional CHD risk factors and treat the inflammation that causes RA itself is necessary and has been found to be effective in treating the RA as well as in reducing the risk of CHD.

Periodontal Disease. Although far from proven, there appears to be strong association between dental plaque and arterial plaque. Gum disease is the most common inflammatory condition in the world. It is present in up to 75 percent of Americans, 20 percent to 30 percent of whom have relatively severe varieties. One of the largest studies to demonstrate a link between periodontal diseases and CHD followed 10,000 healthy individuals for 14 years. Patients who had baseline excellent oral health had a 10 percent risk of developing CHD. In those with mild gingivitis, the risk was 14 percent. However, in patients with full-blown periodontitis, the risk soared to 32 percent. In patients who had lost all of their teeth from gum infections, there was almost a 50 percent chance that they would develop CHD.

Dental plaque is due to a buildup of bacteria on the surfaces of teeth and gums. The associated arterial plaque appears to result not directly from bacteria, but rather from the heightened level of inflammation in the body that occurs when it is constantly fighting off invasive bacteria in the mouth. Patients with periodontal disease have elevated levels of the inflammatory markers CRP and Lp-PLA$_2$. Both substances have been intimately associated with development of arterial plaque. Patients with periodontal disease have been shown to have early plaque in their carotid and coronary arteries as well as endothelial dysfunction more frequently than individuals with good dental hygiene. Conversely, patients treated for periodontal disease show improvement in their level of arterial plaque and their endothelial function, as well as in their levels of CRP and other inflammatory markers.

Chapter 6

Cardiovascular Risk Assessment:
Real Science or Merely Educated Guessing?

IDENTIFYING INDIVIDUALS WHO already have, or are at risk for developing atherosclerosis is both a significant public health and personal health care challenge. This is because atherosclerosis is very prevalent, is usually silent in its early stages and often takes years to develop before it results in symptoms. However, when it is identified early, treatment can not only prevent further progression, it can also result in the lessening of plaque. This process is commonly known as regression of atherosclerosis.

Making the early detection of atherosclerosis of even more importance is the fact that in many instances the first symptom of atherosclerosis may result in death or permanent disability. In more than 25 percent of patients, their first presentation of CHD (coronary heart disease) is a fatal MI or sudden death, with or without an MI. In those who suffer an initial stroke, the mortality rate within the first year following the stroke is 20 percent, and many patients have permanent and significant disability. Thus, early identification and treatment of atherosclerosis can also be lifesaving, life-prolonging and life-preserving.

The most accurate tests to diagnose and detect atherosclerosis are usually expensive, potentially invasive and carry the potential for being time-consuming and potentially risky. Thus, the approach to early diagnosis involves the concept of screening. Cardiovascular screening means that patients undergo relatively inexpensive, simple and safe testing to determine who may be at a higher statistical risk for atherosclerosis. Patients who are identified to be at a higher risk are then referred for more sophisticated testing.

This concept is no different from screening methods for various types of cancer. In breast cancer, a family history or abnormal breast self-examination warrants a mammogram. In colon cancer, the detection of traces of blood in a stool specimen using a Hemoccult card or an abnormal rectal examination leads to colonoscopy. In prostate cancer, an abnormal prostate rectal exam or high prostate-specific antigen (PSA) level in the blood leads to prostate ultrasound and biopsy.

The recommendations for screening are not static but evolve based upon scientific studies as well as changes in the costs and risks associated with screening and follow-up testing. For instance, as colonoscopy has become easier, cheaper and safer, it is now recommended for all individuals over the age of 50, instead of only those failing screening. Thus, for patients over the age of 50 years, colonoscopy itself has become a screening tool. As we will see, such evolution is also very much the case in cardiovascular screening and evaluation. There is an increasing momentum toward the use of simple, inexpensive and safe, noninvasive tests that can directly visualize the artery as an adjunct to traditional screening methods.

In the individual without symptoms, traditional cardiovascular screening typically incorporates the major cardiovascular risk factors identified in the patient's medical history and a fasting blood analysis of a lipid profile to measure cardiovascular risk. Recall that a lipid profile is performed on a fasting sample of blood to measure total cholesterol, triglycerides, LDL-C and HDL-C. There are a number of screening tools, called risk calculators, which are used to quantify an individual's statistical risk of having or developing cardiovascular disease.

Even if the patient is found to not have cardiovascular disease, an estimation of his or her future cardiovascular risk can help to set lipid goals for treatment to prevent CHD. Discussed in the next chapter, these goals are scientifically and statistically validated, such that when achieved they are proven to lower the risk of an individual developing atherosclerosis in the future. In this chapter, we will discuss the screening tools for the detection and follow-up of atherosclerosis.

Keep in mind that CHD screening guidelines and risk-assessment methods are best applied to large populations of patients. They have significant public health value, but they may be quite inadequate when used for a given individual to precisely define his or her statistical risk of developing CHD or clinical events such as an MI or a stroke.

Traditional Screening Methods for Risk Assessment

It is extremely rare to find a patient with CHD without any risk factors. Risk factors tend to cluster in individuals, and clinical events (heart attack, stroke, etc.) are usually the consequence of a moderate elevation of several risk factors rather than a single risk factor. In most individuals, the risk associated with a particular risk factor is also proportional to the severity of the risk factor. Any increasing severity—whether it is a higher level of LDL-C, more body weight, higher blood pressure, more severe diabetes, or greater cigarette consumption—increases the likelihood that CHD exists. In most instances, the risk associated with additional major risk factors increases exponentially and not geometrically. Risk calculators take the major risk factors and incorporate them into validated statistical models to provide estimates of future cardiovascular risk in patients who do not have known CHD.

Using traditional risk factors in screening to assess the future risk of CHD events in an individual has several limitations. First and foremost, they are only statistical estimates. In other words, they represent only educated guesses about the likelihood that you have or will develop CHD. Thus, even if your risk of CHD is low, it will never be zero. There will always be individuals who develop CHD, and its serious consequences of MI, CVA and death, who are found to be at low risk.

As an example, currently 50 million people in the United States are estimated to be at low risk for CHD using the Framingham Risk Scoring (FRS) method of traditional risk screening. By the definition of low risk, one percent to ten percent of these individuals will develop CHD in the next ten years. This translates into between 500,000 to five million "low risk" people who would still develop CHD. Furthermore, we know that in 25 percent of all individuals with CHD, their first presentation is a fatal MI or sudden death. This would then project to a staggering number of between 125,000 and 1.25 million individuals deemed to be at low risk, who, over a ten-year period, would experience the most devastating consequences of CHD! Even more troubling is that the worldwide statistics are worse.

A second limitation is that risk screening has not been validated to evaluate treatment effects. What this means is that if one is found to be at moderate risk for CHD, and is treated, ostensibly to lower the risk, there is no sound information to support an accurate estimate of one's future risk for CHD once the CHD risk factors have been lowered.

There are other significant limitations to conventional CHD risk-screening. No screening method incorporates all possible CHD risk factors. For instance, well-known risk factors of the type we discussed in the last chapter, such as psychological stress, kidney disease, diet and activity habits and rheumatoid arthritis, are not present in any risk calculator. Furthermore, no screening method permits measures of disease severity to be included. CHD risk calculators contain no provisions to distinguish an individual with mild hypertension from one with severe hypertension, or one who is slightly overweight with a BMI of 26 kg/m² from one who is morbidly obese with a BMI of 40 kg/m². These considerations make CHD risk estimates much less valuable for individuals who want to know their specific CHD risk, and much more valuable for public health policy makers and health and life insurance companies.

NCEP Guidelines. The U.S. National Institutes of Health developed the National Cholesterol Education Program (NCEP) guidelines for the evaluation and management of lipid disorders. They are updated periodically by experts in the field, known as the Adult Treatment Panel. These are the guidelines that are followed in the United States by most health care providers, professional societies and the health care industry in general. The most recent update is the third since the NCEP was formed and is thus called Adult Treatment Panel Report III (ATP III).

ATP III indentifies five risk categories based upon CHD risk factors: low risk, moderate risk, moderately-high risk, high risk and very high risk. The major CHD risk factors considered in the NCEP/ATP III initial evaluation of risk are listed in **table 6.1**.

Table 6.1
ATP III Major Cardiovascular Risk Factors

Cigarette Smoking
Hypertension; BP ≥ 140/90 or on BP treatment
Low HDL; < 40 mg/dL
**Family History of premature CHD; First degree relatives with CHD (parents
   or siblings with CHD at or below the ages of 55 if Male or 65 if female)**
Age; Men ≥ 45, Women ≥ 55 years of age

If an individual has zero or one of these risk factors shown in **table 6.1**, he or she is considered to be at low risk, with an estimated likelihood of developing CHD of well below ten percent over the following ten years. Remarkably, since neither total cholesterol nor LDL-C level is considered in the NCEP/ATP III initial evaluation of risk, it is possible to classify a person in a low-risk category no matter what their total cholesterol or LDL-C values. Therein lays just one of the flaws in such risk assessment.

If a person has two or more of these risk factors, the ATP III calls for the further evaluation of CHD risk categories based upon the Framingham Risk Score (FRS), further discussed below. Lipid levels are an important component of risk assessment in the FRS. Risk categories derived from the FRS include low, intermediate and high and are also based upon the likelihood of a person developing CHD over the next ten years. In ATP III, an FRS of less than ten percent indicates a moderate risk of CHD, and an FRS of ten to twenty percent indicates a moderately high risk of CHD.

In the ATP III, high risk is assigned if the FRS is above 20 percent. In addition to a high-risk classification based upon the FRS, the presence of established CHD, symptomatic carotid disease, PVD (peripheral vascular disease) or an AAA (abdominal aortic aneurysm) will also result in a high-risk classification. Also, CHD risk equivalents, such as diabetes or chronic kidney disease, will place a person in the high-risk category. Finally, an individual with an FRS of 10–20 percent, but with an elevated CRP level as evidence of vascular inflammation is also considered high risk for CHD.

The final category is very high risk. Very high risk patients are those who have had a recent MI or episode of angina requiring hospitalization. This is also known by the term ACS, meaning acute coronary syndrome. Also patients with established CHD or CVD (cerebrovascular disease), who also have multiple active risk factors for CHD that are severe and poorly controlled, such as metabolic syndrome, diabetes or ongoing tobacco use qualify as very high risk individuals. The NCEP/ATP III risk categories and risk-stratification guidelines are presented in **table 6.2.**

Table 6.2
NCEP Risk Stratification Guidelines

Risk category	Criteria
Low	One or fewer Major ATP III risk factors (see Table 6.1)
Moderate	Two or more Major ATP III risk factors, and a FRS <10%
Moderately High	Two or more Major ATP III risk factors, and a FRS of 10-20%
High	Two or more Major ATP III risk factors, and a FRS of >20%, or a FRS of 10-20% with a CRP > 2.0 mg/L, or Established CHD, PVD, AAA, CVD, or CHD risk equivalents (diabetes or CKD)
Very High	Acute CHD; acute coronary syndrome/MI, or Chronic CHD/CVD, with multiple active risk factors (diabetes, smoking, metabolic syndrome)

Definitions;
   ATP III = Adult Treatment Panel III, National Cholesterol Education Program (NCEP)
   FRS = Framingham Risk Score
   CRP = C-reactive protein, by high-sensitivity (hs) method
   CHD = coronary heart disease, established by any clinical or imaging method
   PVD = peripheral vascular disease
   AAA= abdominal aortic aneurysm
   CVD= cerebrovascular disease ($\geq$ 50% stenosis in a carotid artery)
   CKD= chronic kidney disease (serum creatnine level of $\geq$ 1.5 mg/dL)

Framingham Risk Score. We have previously discussed some of the important clinical data that has come from the Framingham Heart Study. Initiated in 1948, this database of patients in Framingham, Massachusetts, continues to provide valuable epidemiological data about CHD. One of the most important contributions of Framingham and its researchers is the risk-prediction functions derived from the database of patients. The first risk calculator was introduced in the 1960s. The most current risk calculator is known as the revised Framingham Risk Score (FRS), a significant component of the treatment recommendations for risk modification in the NCEP guidelines.

The FRS uses the components of (1) age, (2) sex, (3) total cholesterol, (4) smoking status, (5) HDL-C and (6) systolic BP to derive an estimate of the risk that a given individual will develop CHD within the next ten years. Each of the above criteria is assigned points in the statistical model that influence the estimate of ten-year risk. In the FRS, a ten-year risk of less than ten percent is considered low, ten to twenty percent is intermediate, and greater than 20 percent is considered high risk. If an individual has two or more ATP III risk factors, the calculation of an FRS provides additional value in his or her risk assessment.

> **Illumination:** If you know your blood pressure readings and lipid values, you can calculate your own FRS using one of the many available online calculators, such as this one sponsored by the National Heart, Lung, and Blood Institute:
>
> http://hp2010.nhlbihin.net/atpiii/calculator.asp?usertype=prof

The FRS is a statistically validated algorithm and thus has value in the population in which it was studied. This is another criticism of risk calculators like the FRS. The majority of patients studied to derive the FRS were middle-aged, white, middle-class men. In a study of offspring of patients enrolled in the original Framingham studies, the FRS was shown to under-estimate CHD risk in younger (under 50 years of age) individuals and in women. Another criticism is that the FRS does not take into account many other important CHD risk factors, including diabetes, metabolic syndrome, markers of inflammation, family history, kidney disease, body weight, physical activity, stress and other lipid parameters, as well as many emerging risk factors.

Other Risk Calculators. Since CHD risk appears to be specific to the population in which it is studied, improved risk estimates may be possible using data unique to the population in question. In Europe, the SCORE risk charts are widely used, and may be a better predictor of CHD death than the FRS. However, for risk estimates, they perform better in European populations than in Americans, Asians or Africans. Risk calculators from Asian countries likewise appear to be better at evaluating risk estimates in Asians than in Western societies. The QRISK2 score from the United Kingdom makes an attempt to be more widely applicable by including ethnicity, BMI, family history of CHD and social status.

One particularly useful new risk calculator appears to be the Reynolds Risk Score (RRS). The RRS was introduced in 2007 after being validated in a ten-year follow-up of a cohort of 25,000 women who participated in the Women's Health Study. Two new variables not found in the FRS were discovered to be significant and incorporated into this new score: a parental history of premature CHD and an assessment of inflammation using the blood test for C-reactive protein (CRP).

Illumination: You can calculate your RRS using the tool found online at the following link:

http://www.reynoldsriskscore.org/

Using the RRS scoring system, 40–50 percent of women previously estimated by the FRS to be intermediate risk, were reclassified as either low or high risk (**table 6.3**). Subsequent studies show that the RRS is also valuable for men. Since it is impossible to know which risk calculator is actually correct, the discovery that there are frequent discrepancies between the risk estimates by these highly validated CHD statistical risk calculators has further intensified the debate as to whether such calculators have significant value in a given individual's risk assessment.

Table 6.3
Disparity Between FRS and RRS
Risk Stratification

Risk Parameter	Value	10-year risk by FRS	10-year risk by RRS
Gender	Female		
Age	72		
BP (systolic)	145 mmHg		
Diabetes?	No		
Smoker?	Yes	4.9%	23.2%
Total Cholesterol	216 mg/dL		
HDL-C	82 mg/dL		
hs-CRP	7.7 mg/L		
Family History CHD	Yes		

In the example shown, the same risk parameter values in this individual yielded vastly different assessments of 10-year risk by the FRS and the RRS methods.

FRS = Framingham Risk Score
RRS = Reynolds Risk Score
BP = Blood Pressure
HDL-C = HDL Cholesterol
hs-CRP = C-reactive protein measured using the high-sensitivity method
CHD = Coronary Heart Disease

CHD Risk Equivalents. Certain CHD risk factors pose such a high risk for CHD that they are considered CHD risk equivalents. This means that patients with these risks should be considered as already having a diagnosis of CHD, even though they may not have had any symptoms or clinical consequences. Such patients are classified as high risk. We have already noted that diabetes is in this category. Some experts also consider chronic kidney disease (CKD) to be in this category. Patients with these diseases often have other CHD risk factors, such as hypertension and lipid abnormalities. When large populations of these patients are studied, their prognoses and outcomes are no different than those of patients who already carry a diagnosis of CHD. Therefore, it is recommended that these patients be treated as aggressively in management of their risk factors and lipid abnormalities as patients who already have CHD.

Cardiovascular Imaging Methods for Screening

Atherosclerosis is a disease that affects the blood vessels of the heart and circulatory system. It is therefore completely reasonable to believe that a direct examination of blood vessels would then be the most direct way to determine the presence and extent of atherosclerosis. However, most techniques that look directly at blood vessels with sufficient accuracy to visualize plaque require invasive examinations and thus carry risks such as injury to the blood vessels, allergic reactions to iodine dye and radiation exposure, to name only a few. Furthermore, such examinations are expensive, time-consuming and may be painful. Finally, traditional techniques that examine coronary arteries do not have the ability to accurately detect the very early stages of atherosclerosis.

Recently, several types of examinations that provide images of blood vessels have shown the ability to overcome these limitations. In an effort to promote the adoption of direct imaging of blood vessels, in 2006, the Society for Heart Attack Prevention and Eradication (SHAPE) began to promote a set of guidelines that incorporate imaging tests with traditional screening methods to improve the success of identifying at-risk individuals. The SHAPE guidelines highlight one of the problems with traditional risk-screening calculators, such as the Framingham Risk Score—namely, that they are based on population studies, and health care providers are required to extrapolate the data to the individual patient. By examining the blood vessels in the specific individual, imaging tests provide information that is unique to that patient and their arteries.

The first SHAPE guidelines established standards for implementation of scientifically proven atherosclerosis tests to detect subclinical disease in the coronary and carotid arteries. Two types of examinations, carotid ultrasound and coronary CAT scans, are recommended by the SHAPE guidelines to be incorporated into the routine screening for all asymptomatic men age 45 to 75 years and asymptomatic women age 55 to 75 years, except for those defined as very low risk because of the absence of known ATP III risk factors. The SHAPE guidelines also became the basis for the Texas

Heart Attack Prevention Bill, signed into law in Texas in 2009. In 2010, the American Heart Association and the American College of Cardiology recognized the value of the same screening methods in their updated guidelines for risk assessment in asymptomatic individuals. In theory, by combining standard risk assessment methods with imaging tests, we can even further refine risk estimates, as well as have a tool to directly evaluate the effects of treatment on the health of a specific patient's arteries.

Still, several limitations to the widespread use of these newer techniques still exist. One such limitation is access to the tests, since they require specialized equipment and the expertise of a physician to be properly interpreted. A second limitation is that such examinations are usually not covered by most health insurance plans as screening tests. Nevertheless, there is increasing enthusiasm for the use of such examinations in properly selected individuals who have no symptoms of atherosclerosis. Also, a significant decline in costs of these exams has made them affordable to many individuals even without significant insurance coverage. This area remains an active area of interest as well as controversy in public health and cardiovascular disease prevention.

Carotid Ultrasound. The technique of carotid ultrasound uses reflected sound waves to generate pictures of the carotid arteries. The technique uses the same type of ultrasound instrument that is used to obtain images of a fetus in the womb. The technique is completely safe, painless, simple and noninvasive, as well as relatively inexpensive and widely available.

The examination has such high resolution and accuracy that it is possible to measure the thickness of the two interior layers of the carotid artery, the intima and media. You will recall that these two layers are where the earliest stages of plaque growth occur. Thus, carotid ultrasound can detect the earliest changes in the artery, even before the development of full-blown plaque. The measurement of the thickness of the visible layers of the carotid arterial intima and media is known as the cIMT (carotid intimal-medial thickness).

The technology for the measurement of cIMT has been around since 1986. It is not available for the coronary arteries of the heart, but it is well recognized and validated that changes in the cIMT closely correspond to the same changes inside the heart's coronary arteries, as well as in the brain's cerebral blood vessels, the aorta and the leg blood vessels. Furthermore, an increase in cIMT is associated with adverse cardiovascular events such as MI, CVA and death. Since the technique is so simple, it can be repeated periodically to monitor the effectiveness of treatment to prevent or reverse atherosclerosis.

Coronary CAT Scanning. Computerized axial tomography (CAT) scans have been widely used for a variety of medical imaging needs. Recent improvements in the technique have greatly increased resolution, lowered radiation exposure and reduced costs. The most widely used CHD screening method by CAT scanning is called the coronary calcium score (CCS). Like carotid ultrasound, this technique is also noninvasive, painless and widely available. Unlike carotid ultrasound, the examination has the capability to look at the coronary arteries in the heart. However, the scan does not provide the same detail of the blood vessel wall as in an ultrasound exam. Instead, the CCS exam looks for the presence of calcium in the artery wall and can actually provide a quantitative estimate of the relative amount of accumulated calcium. You will recall that calcium deposits in the wall of the coronary artery frequently accompany the development of atherosclerosis.

> **Illumination:** The original CCS was developed in 1998 by Dr. Arthur Agatson, who is also famous for developing the South Beach Diet. The CCS corresponds closely with early plaque development. Any CCS above zero is considered indicative of the presence of atherosclerosis. However, a score of 0–100 is considered low risk, 100–400 intermediate risk, 400–1,000 high risk and above 1,000 highest risk.

The ability of CAT scan imaging to detect calcium in the coronary arteries varies by patient sex and race. Usually calcium is more readily detected in white men than in women or any other racial subgroup. This may be a function of the incidence of atherosclerosis or, alternatively, it may reflect that calcium deposits do not always accompany atherosclerosis in all individuals. We know that soft plaque typically does not contain calcium, whereas hard plaque usually does. This may be a limitation of the CCS as a screening tool. However, research has shown that the CCS provides additional value to the FRS in identifying high-risk patients.

Cardiac Magnetic Resonance Imaging. The use of carotid imaging to measure cIMT and CAT scans to gauge CCS is available in many communities and is part of the SHAPE guidelines. There are, in fact, newer techniques that offer even more promise as screening arterial imaging methods. One such technique is cardiac magnetic resonance imaging (MRI). Many local health centers now have MRI equipment. MRI uses no radiation and is safe, simple, noninvasive and painless. MRI provides a direct exam of the coronary artery. It has been shown capable of providing exquisite detail of plaque in the coronary arteries. Not only can it potentially provide accurate estimates of the amount of plaque present, it can look at calcium deposits in the plaque as well as the fibrous capsule overlying the plaque. The major obstacles to its widespread use include cost, access to the equipment properly configured for coronary artery imaging and ongoing discussion on the validation of its utility and accuracy. Cardiac MRI offers great promise and potential as a screening tool for the early diagnosis of CHD.

Chapter 7

Blood Testing in the Assessment of Cardiovascular Risk:

Establishing Goals of Therapy to Prevent, Treat and Reverse Atherosclerosis

RISK ASSESSMENT AND screening discussed in the previous chapter guides the strategies that are used to prevent, treat and reverse CHD (coronary heart disease). First and foremost, the treatment and control of all modifiable risk factors is a goal, no matter what a person's cardiovascular risk is measured to be. Thus, controlling and modifying blood pressure, diabetes, weight, diet, smoking status, stress and any other identified risk factors are core principles in CHD management.

The identification of an individual's CHD (coronary heart disease) risk, whether it is by a risk calculator like the FRS (Framingham Risk Score) or RRS (Reynolds Risk Score), by imaging methods, or by clinical circumstances, helps to determine that person's blood lipid goals. In this chapter, we will review the specific goals and recommendations for the traditional lipid values. We will also discuss the value of some of the other emerging, commonly measured and useful lipid, inflammatory and genetic markers derived from more sophisticated testing methods that may help to further refine and individualize risk assessment and treatment.

A number of lipid components measured in the bloodstream are targets for treatment. This means that there is sound scientific data to support the premise that not only do abnormal levels of these components contribute to atherosclerosis, but treating these abnormalities can retard progression of atherosclerosis as well as induce regression of atherosclerosis. Furthermore, treating these lipid abnormalities may also reduce the likelihood of atherosclerosis-related illnesses like MI and stroke as well as CHD-related death. Some of the most important lipid targets for treatment are discussed in the following sections.

Traditional Lipid Parameters

Most of the lipid parameters discussed below can be measured by simple blood tests. In some tests, the blood needs to be drawn while fasting, but in most cases a non-fasting sample is acceptable. The blood analysis of traditional lipid parameters can be performed by most local laboratories. The value of monitoring blood lipids is recognized by most health insurance plans, and this type of testing is usually covered up to four times a year by most commercial and Medicare insurance plans.

Total Cholesterol. We are all familiar with the notion that we want to control our cholesterol. Historically, the development of the "lipid hypothesis" postulated that elevated cholesterol caused atherosclerosis. It was not too long ago that the U.S. government initiated the public health campaign 'Know Your Number,' in an effort to make our society more conscious about cholesterol.

In fact, knowledge about your level of Total Cholesterol is of almost no value in identifying patients at risk for CHD. Data from the Framingham study has established that patients without CHD are as likely to have Total Cholesterol readings above 200 mg/dL as they are to have readings below 200 mg/dL. Further analysis of this data has indicated that as many as one-third of all coronary heart disease (CHD) events occur in individuals with total cholesterol less than 200 mg/dL. One-half of all heart attack victims have low to moderate total cholesterol levels. Total cholesterol has no predictive value in identifying patients at risk for stroke. Since total cholesterol also includes HDL-C, it does not account for the protective benefit that exists in many patients who have high levels of HDL-C. Observations such as this, as well as an improved understanding of cholesterol metabolism, have helped to refine our concepts of what are harmful and disease-causing lipid levels.

When we perform a standard lipid blood test, the report returns values for Total Cholesterol, LDL-C, HDL-C and triglycerides. For the reasons noted above, the Total Cholesterol is the least useful. Although the NCEP guidelines set cholesterol values of less than 200 mg/dL as desirable, 200–239 mg/dL as borderline high, and above 239 mg/dL as high, the guidelines no longer indicate cholesterol levels as targets of therapy. As noted below, the LDL-C is the more useful value in predicting CHD risk, as well as in the goal of treatment and risk reduction.

LDL Cholesterol. The NCEP guidelines, updated in 2004, indicate that LDL-C is the primary target of therapy in the management of all CHD risk categories. The level of desired LDL-C is based upon the CHD risk determined for a given individual. Recall that risk can be categorized using risk calculators such as FRS as low, intermediate or high. These usually correspond to the risk of developing CHD over a ten-year period of less than ten percent, ten to twenty percent and greater than 20 percent, respectively. Recall also that the NCEP further refines the risk assessments of the FRS by the addition of two additional risk categories. The NCEP LDL-C goals listed, based upon the five CHD risk categories, are noted in **table 7.1.**

Table 7.1
NCEP Lipid Goals

Risk category	LDL-C Target (mg/dL)	Non-HDL-C Target* (mg/dL)	Apo B100 Target (mg/dL)
Low	< 160 (optional <130)	<190	<130
Moderate	< 130 (optional <100)	<160	<110
Moderately High	<100 (optional <70)	<130	<90
High	<100 (optional <70)	<130	<90
Very High	<70	<100	<80

*the Non-HDL-C target is valid if Triglyceride levels are above 150 mg/dL

NCEP = National Cholesterol Education Program
LDL-C = LDL cholesterol
HDL-C = HDL cholesterol
Apo B100 = Apolipoprotein B100 level

The blood level of LDL-C is closely and directly related to the development of CHD. Higher LDL-C levels lead to more atherosclerosis and a higher risk of CHD events such as MI, stroke and sudden death, as well as a need for angioplasty and bypass surgery. Also, a reduction in LDL-C has been shown to not only reduce the occurrence of events, but also cause regression of existing plaque. For every one percent change in LDL-C, there is a one percent change in CHD risk. Thus a 20 percent rise in LDL-C raises CHD risk by 20 percent, and likewise a 20 percent drop will reduce CHD risk by the same amount.

For high-risk and very high-risk patients, an LDL-C of less than 70 mg/dL is considered optimal. Data from numerous clinical studies support this threshold LDL-C as the point at which there is a significant reduction in statistical risk of CHD events. This level is also the LDL-C threshold that is most often associated with plaque regression.

> **Illumination:** There is reason to believe that teleologically an LDL-C of around 70 mg/dL is what nature intended. Most mammals have LDL-C levels of about 70 mg/dL. Human infants at birth have LDL-C levels of about 70 mg/dL. Adults not following western diets and lifestyles maintain LDL-C levels of about 70 mg/dL throughout their lives.

LDL-C in a standard lipid test is a calculated number based upon the levels of measured total cholesterol, HDL-C and triglycerides. This is because the assay for direct LDL-C measurement is quite complicated and cumbersome, and therefore also expensive. In most cases the calculated LDL-C level is accurate. However, in certain situations a directly measured LDL-C determined using advanced lipid testing is more accurate. This is especially true if the blood sample is nonfasting, if triglyceride levels are high, in patients with diabetes or if LDL-C levels are very low.

HDL Cholesterol. Unlike LDL-C, which plays a key role in plaque development, HDL-C protects against plaque development. Many population studies indicate that HDL-C may be an even stronger predictor of CHD than LDL-C. HDL-C has a strong inverse relationship with cardiovascular risk. For every one mg/dL rise in HDL-C, there is a three to four percent lowering of CHD risk, and vice versa. Thus, all else being equal, an individual with an HDL-C level of 50 mg/dL is 40 percent less likely to have CHD than someone with an HDL-C of 40 mg/dL. However, the evidence that raising a given individual's HDL-C will substantially lower that individual's CHD risk remains elusive. Still, in most instances it is considered worthwhile to try to optimize HDL-C.

Since an elevated HDL-C is considered a favorable risk factor, most risk calculators consider an HDL-C 60 mg/dL or higher to reduce CHD risk estimates. An HDL-C level under 40 mg/dL is considered an adverse risk factor for CHD. Even though HDL is highly inherited, it can be affected by certain environmental influences. HDL-C is typically depressed further whenever triglyceride levels are increased. Lack of physical activity, high carbohydrate diets and smoking all depress HDL-C, as do certain medications like anabolic steroids and progestin.

Raising HDL-C is difficult, and HDL-C levels are only modestly altered by typical lipid modification strategies, including diet, exercise and medications. In some individuals, modest alcohol consumption and cessation of cigarette use can have significant favorable effects on HDL-C levels. One reason pre-menopausal women have a lower risk of CHD than men of similar ages is the higher levels of HDL-C in women.

Triglycerides. The fourth and final component that is analyzed in standard lipid testing is the level of triglycerides. Typically, isolated triglyceride elevations are not associated with CHD. The most common genetic disorder causing triglyceride elevations is familial hypertriglyceridemia, which occurs in one to two percent of the population. In this disorder, triglyceride levels are often in excess of 500 mg/dL. However, it is one of the few genetic lipid disorders that are not associated with an increased risk of CHD. In fact, the only lipid disorder for which the NCEP guidelines indicate that LDL-C control is not the primary goal of therapy is when triglyceride levels are above 500 mg/dL. In such individuals, there is a much higher risk of developing pancreatitis than there is a risk of CHD, so the aim of treatment is to lower triglyceride levels prior to therapy directed toward LDL-C.

Unlike LDL-C elevations, which typically occur only due to an increased endogenous LDL synthesis, exogenous saturated fat and cholesterol intake or decreased liver clearance of LDL, there are many more causes for increased triglycerides. These include: (1) genetic disorders like familial hypertriglyceridemia, (2) medications like steroids, oral estrogens and diuretics, (3) medical conditions like diabetes, metabolic syndrome, kidney disorders, thyroid disorders, liver disease and pregnancy, and (4) lifestyle conditions, such as obesity, high carbohydrate diets, alcoholism and cigarette smoking.

When triglyceride levels are associated with low HDL-C, as is often the case, or when triglyceride elevations occur in certain populations of subjects such as diabetics, post-menopausal women and individuals with metabolic syndrome, the risk of CHD does appear to be increased. In such patients, triglyceride levels above 150 mg/dL can cause a shift in LDL particles to the smaller, denser variety and hence result in an increased number of LDL particles that are more atherogenic. Elevated triglyceride levels also lead to higher levels of remnant lipoproteins like VLDL and IDL, which, by virtue of containing the Apo B100 molecule, are also atherogenic. Thus, it is recommended that triglyceride levels be maintained below 150 mg/dL. Indeed in such patients, elevated triglycerides appear to affect statistical risk in much the same way as LDL-C and HDL-C levels do. Women appear to be more sensitive to triglyceride elevations than do men.

Alert! For every 100 mg/dL change in triglycerides (either up or down), there is a same-direction and concomitant 14 percent change in the risk of CHD events for men—and an astounding 40 percent change in the risk of CHD for women!

Advanced Lipid Testing

Advanced lipid testing is usually reserved for patients who have abnormalities in the standard lipid blood tests. It is also performed in individuals who have a strong family history of CHD, significant and/or multiple nonlipid risk factors, established CHD or those who are on medications for treatment of lipid disorders. Advanced lipid testing is more sophisticated and more expensive than standard lipid tests. However, not only does it provide more information specific to your lipid issues, it can also help guide more specific and individualized treatment.

The analysis of advanced lipid parameters requires specialized analysis that is available in only a few select laboratories. In this case, the blood specimen can be drawn in your local laboratory and is usually shipped to the specialized laboratory that has the necessary equipment and standardized measurement methods. It is more expensive than standard lipid testing, yet many patients and health care providers are not aware that the majority of the cost of this type of advanced testing is usually covered by most Medicare and other health insurance plans.

Advanced lipid testing helps to further refine the risk estimates that are obtained from standard lipid testing. As we have previously discussed, the results of standard lipid tests that are used in CHD risk calculators are poorly suited to guide assessment of individualized risk and treatment. Indeed, traditional lipid risk factors for atherosclerosis account for only 40 percent of premature CHD. In some cases, advanced lipid testing may actually avoid the unnecessary use of medications in those patients who, by the analysis of the standard lipid parameters, would otherwise qualify for medications.

Apolipoprotein B100. Many studies indicate that the strongest predictor of CHD risk is not LDL-C, but instead is apolipoprotein B100 (Apo B100). Recall that the Apo B100 molecule is attached not only to every LDL particle but also to every non-HDL lipoprotein, including VLDL and IDL particles. It appears to be the primary mediator of lipid deposition into arterial plaque. There is more Apo B100 when there are more LDL particles present in the bloodstream. In certain individuals, LDL-C may be relatively low compared to their Apo B100 levels, since their LDL particles are smaller. However, these individuals still carry a significant CHD risk.

As with LDL-C, Apo B100 desirable target levels are also based upon CHD risk (**table 7.1**). For most individuals, an Apo B100 of greater than 120 mg/dL is considered high risk, and less than 80 mg/dL is considered optimal, especially if the patient is already in the very high-risk CHD category. Many experts, including those at the American Diabetes Association and the American College of Cardiology, suggest that Apo B100 replace

LDL-C as the target for therapy. Many guidelines for treatment of lipid disorders, including those used in Canada and Europe, support Apo B100 levels instead of LDL-C as the therapeutic target.

Non-HDL Cholesterol. Non-HDL cholesterol is simply the measured
amount of cholesterol contained in all lipid particles except the HDL
particles. Since the HDL particle is protective, this measurement reflects all of
the cholesterol present only in the particles that can cause atherosclerosis.
Non-HDL cholesterol is a calculated number derived from a simple
mathematical formula: *Non-HDL cholesterol = Total Cholesterol – HDL cholesterol*

This measurement is especially useful in patients who have high levels
of triglycerides, since the elevated triglycerides contribute to the formation
of more VLDL and IDL particles. Both VLDL and IDL are also atherogenic and are known as remnant lipoproteins, as they represent an intermediary step toward ultimate conversion into LDL particles.

As one might expect, the non-HDL cholesterol typically corresponds
to the level of Apo B100, since every non-HDL particle contains one molecule of Apo B100. The non-HDL cholesterol level also corresponds to the
number of LDL particles. Since non-HDL cholesterol can be measured
from the standard lipid panel, and Apo B100 and LDL particle number
measurements require advanced lipid testing, the non-HDL cholesterol
reading is easier, quicker and cheaper to obtain.

The desired non-HDL cholesterol target level is linked to the LDL-C
target, as defined by the NCEP risk guidelines noted in **table 7.1**. The non-
HDL goals are invoked when triglyceride levels are greater than 150 mg/dL
and after the LDL-C goal for the specific risk category has been achieved.
For each risk category, the non-HDL target is simply 30 mg/dL higher than
the corresponding LDL-C target level.

LDL Particle Size, Density and Number. Recall that LDL particles
are present in a continuum of size and density. Usually, when LDL particles
are smaller and denser, there is also an increase in the number of LDL particles. As we have previously discussed, in Chapter four, when this occurs,
the measured LDL-C may not reflect the true pathogenic potential for

atherosclerosis, since the number and size of the LDL particles is a stronger influence on plaque formation than the LDL-C level (recall the analogy of the cars on the highway from Chapter four: more cars has a greater effect on causing an arterial blockage than more passengers).

LDL particle analysis requires advanced lipid testing. This blood exam provides much more information about CHD risk as well as success of treatment for prevention and reversal of atherosclerosis than the standard lipid panel. The examination is well worth doing in patients who are being aggressively monitored and treated, since having LDL particles that are plentiful, small and dense is much worse than just having high LDL-C. Having dense LDL means two to four times more risk for development of CHD than a high level of LDL-C. Also, regression of plaque occurs much more commonly in patients who are able to reduce the amount of small, dense LDL rather than just LDL-C alone.

The evaluation of particle number and size is particularly important when triglyceride levels are high and/or HDL-C levels are low. In both of these circumstances, there is a very prominent disconnection between LDL-C and the number of circulating LDL particles. The LDL-C level may be quite normal or near normal, when in fact the circulating numbers of LDL particles (and Apo B100) are, in fact, quite high.

The Multi-Ethnic Study of Atherosclerosis (MESA) followed nearly 6,000 individuals without known CHD. Subjects who had high levels of circulating LDL particles but normal LDL-C levels had a three-fold higher risk of CHD events than those with low levels of circulating LDL particles and high levels of LDL-C. The landmark Framingham Offspring Study, which followed more than 3,000 men and women over 15 years, found similar results. The LDL particle number was twice as strongly associated with increased CHD risks as was LDL-C. The non-HDL cholesterol was also better than LDL-C in predicting CHD risk, but was not as good as the LDL particle number. In fact, patients with a low LDL-C but a high LDL particle number were twice as likely to have CHD events as patients with a high LDL-C and a low LDL particle number.

> **Alert!** One very important finding of the Framingham Offspring Study was that in individuals with low LDL-C levels that occur either naturally or especially through LDL-lowering therapy, LDL particle numbers may still be elevated, since often these patients develop cholesterol-depleted LDL particles, which can contribute to an underestimation of both LDL and CHD risk when measured by LDL-C levels. Therefore, if CHD risk is significantly elevated or the individual is receiving treatment to lower LDL-C, a measurement of LDL particle number is a much more accurate predictor of further CHD risk.

As we previously said, small, dense LDL particles more easily penetrate the endothelium and enter the arterial wall. They are more easily trapped by the web-like matrix of protein and sugar molecules called proteoglycans in the arterial wall and oxidized, which makes them more susceptible to being swallowed up by the scavenger macrophages, which turn LDL-C into cholesterol plaque. Most of the time, having a predominance of small, dense LDL particles is associated with having a higher absolute number of LDL particles. This also corresponds with a higher level of Apo B100, since each Apo B100 molecule requires an LDL particle.

The most desirable LDL density pattern is to have more than 70 percent of the LDL particles in the large, buoyant category and less than 30 percent in the small, dense category. Since lipoproteins particles are so small, their levels are measured in units of nanomoles (nmol), and expressed as a concentration in the bloodstream. The desirable number for total LDL particles is less than 1,000 nmol/L (nanomoles/Liter).

HDL Particle Size, Density and Number. The primary protein component of HDL particles is apolipoprotein A (Apo A). This apolipoprotein distinguishes the HDL from LDL particle, which contains Apo B100 as its primary protein component. As with LDL, the family of HDL particles also occurs along a continuum of size and density. HDLs can also be divided into the smaller, denser particles and the larger, buoyant particles. The larger, spherical HDL particles are more efficient "garbage trucks," as they more effectively remove cholesterol from cells and take it back to the liver. In the HDL class of particles, the most protective, largest and lightest types of HDL particles are called HDL-2, among which the subcategory of HDL-2_b particles are the most beneficial.

In one study of nearly 1,200 men, those with the highest levels of the large HDL-2_b particles had an almost 80 percent reduced risk of CHD compared to those with the lowest levels of HDL-2_b. On the other hand, the smaller, denser HDL of the type known as HDL-3_b may actually be associated with an increased risk of CHD. While HDL-C can be measured using standard lipid testing, the measurement of HDL subtypes requires advanced lipid testing.

Medications and non-pharmacologic therapies that aim to affect HDL vary considerably in their effectiveness as well as in their relative effect on the total number of HDL particles, HDL subtypes and HDL-C. Therefore, knowledge of HDL particle number and subtypes can help guide treatment programs. The desired level of all HDL-2 subtypes is an absolute value of greater than 10 mg/dL, or a relative value of greater than 20 percent of all the HDL subtypes. The desirable number of total HDL particles is greater than 7,000 nmol/L and HDL-2_b particles above 1,400 nmol/L.

Lipoprotein (a). Lipoprotein (a), also known as Lp(a), consists of a small, dense LDL particle attached to an additional apolipoprotein called apo(a). When the LDL particle is so modified, it becomes even more atherogenic than it already is.

Illumination: It is estimated that the cholesterol content of the Lp(a) particles is ten times as atherogenic as that of the typical LDL particle.

Since Lp(a) contains the Apo B100 apolipoprotein, it is an atherogenic particle. However, the apo(a) apolipoprotein also confers to the Lp(a) particle the property of also promoting blood clotting, also known as being thrombogenic. The apo(a) complex attached to the LDL particle has a corkscrew shape. This is very similar to what is found in the blood clot dissolving factor plasminogen. The similarity of Lp(a) to plasminogen makes naturally occurring plasminogen less effective. This means the LDL particle to which apo(a) is attached can help to induce blood clots inside the blood vessel. Hence, Lp(a) is known as the "heart attack protein." Many experts believe that Lp(a) may be the so-called missing link between atherosclerosis and thrombosis.

In patients judged to be at high risk for atherosclerosis, elevated Lp(a) is found in nearly 40 percent of individuals, compared to only 14 percent of patients judged to be at low risk. High levels of Lp(a), those above 30 mg/dL, are strongly associated with a higher risk of CHD, stroke and peripheral vascular disease. The desirable level is less than 10 mg/dL. Lp(a) is found in elevated levels especially in younger patients with CHD and in some ethnic groups, and so may have a significant genetic control. It is also elevated in diabetics, and in those diabetics with high Lp(a) levels, there is nearly a four-fold higher risk of CHD compared to diabetics with normal Lp(a) levels. The best way to lower Lp(a) is to lower LDL-C. Some treatments that lower LDL-C lower Lp(a) better than others, so knowing the Lp(a) may help guide which would be the best treatment for reduction of both Lp(a) and LDL-C.

Oxidized LDL. Oxidized LDL is the atherogenic form of LDL. The oxidation process takes place in the arterial wall after the LDL particle enters through the endothelium into the intimal layer of the artery. The oxidation of LDL leads to its uptake into macrophages and the subsequent development of the cholesterol plaque. Oxidized LDL is found primarily in plaque and not in normal arteries.

A number of biomarkers that reflect oxidative stress in the artery have been evaluated as a way to identify patients who are at a higher risk for or are actually developing plaque. One such marker is the actual level of oxidized LDL. This can be measured in the bloodstream and theoretically reflects the amount of oxidized LDL that is present in the arterial wall. The major problem in using markers of oxidative stress is that there is a relatively short-lived impact of acute oxidative stress. Thus, being able to detect the rapid biological changes that occur in the arterial wall by using a blood test is a significant challenge.

Nevertheless, a number of clinical studies show that elevated levels of oxidized LDL are better able to distinguish patients with CHD from those without, compared to total cholesterol levels and even LDL-C levels. When combined with the level of HDL-C as a ratio of oxidized LDL:HDL-C, the measurement has even better discriminative power to identify patients at risk for CHD. The levels of oxidized LDL, measured in units per liter (U/L), can help categorize a patient's relative CHD risk. An oxidized LDL level of less than 45 U/L is considered low risk, 45–59 U/L moderate risk, 60–79 U/L high risk, and above 79 U/L very high risk.

Inflammatory Markers

Inflammation in the blood vessel wall is a key component of the atherosclerosis process. Markers of inflammation are increasingly being used as indicators of atherosclerosis risk. These markers may not only identify persons at higher risk of developing or who have developed atherosclerosis, but they may also better identify those individuals in whom atherosclerosis may imminently cause serious illnesses such as MI and stroke than traditional lipid parameters. Finally, treatments that result in a reduction in inflammation as noted by an improvement in the level of inflammatory markers appear to also be associated with a reduction in the risk of serious illnesses. In this section, we will discuss two of the most commonly used markers that are used to identify patients with vascular inflammation.

C-Reactive Protein. C-reactive protein (CRP) is implicated as a key participant in the inflammatory process that leads to atherosclerosis. The CRP molecule has been shown to activate inflammation at many levels. Beyond its role in inflammation, it also is involved in nearly all other aspects of plaque formation. Evidence supports its role in causing endothelial dysfunction. It has pro-thrombotic properties that help facilitate blood clotting as well as vasoconstrictive properties that can make the artery more likely to spasm and narrow.

In addition to playing a significant role in atherosclerosis, it is also a marker for patients at risk for, or who already have atherosclerosis. It is present in the blood of patients who have CHD, as well as those who develop MI and stroke, more frequently and at higher levels than in those who do not have CHD. Multiple clinical studies support the value of CRP as an independent risk factor for CHD. The Physicians' Health Study (PHS) of nearly 15,000 men without previous heart disease, who were studied for a nine-year period, found that patients with the highest levels of CRP had a 5.3 times increased risk of having their first MI, compared to those patients having the lowest levels of CRP. Remarkably, the Women's Health Study (WHS) of 25,000 women, studied for a ten-year period, showed almost the same exact results. As noted in the last chapter, the CRP level has been found to be of additional benefit when added to risk assessment using the risk calculator of the Reynolds Risk Score.

Since CRP is found in higher levels with other diseases that cause chronic and acute inflammatory responses, the proper assessment for the purposes of identifying heart risk is done using a technique known as a high-sensitivity assay. This permits the detection of very low levels of CRP, or high-sensitivity CRP (hs-CRP). Levels of hs-CRP less than one mg/L identify patients at low risk for CHD, levels of one to three mg/L indicate intermediate risk, and levels above three mg/L are considered high risk.

Lipoprotein-Associated Phospholipase A2 Complex. The lipoprotein-associated phospholipase A2 complex (Lp-PLA$_2$) is a molecule that circulates in the bloodstream primarily attached to the LDL particle. It helps to facilitate oxidation of the LDL particle as well as an inflammatory response to the LDL particle once it penetrates the arterial wall. The Lp-PLA$_2$ molecule is found in abundance in the arterial wall at the sites of plaque rupture. In the same way that Lp(a) may be the missing link between atherosclerosis and thrombosis, many experts consider Lp-PLA$_2$ to be the missing link between oxidation and inflammation in the arterial wall.

Lp-PLA$_2$ levels can be measured in the blood, and they help identify patients with vascular inflammation. The Lp-PLA$_2$ may be better than the hs-CRP exam because, unlike CRP, Lp-PLA$_2$ is more specific to inflammation confined to the blood vessel and not other causes of inflammation in the body. An elevated level of Lp-PLA$_2$ also identifies patients at increased risk for plaque rupture and thus development of MI or stroke. Elevated levels of Lp-PLA$_2$ identify patients at a two-fold increased risk for cardiovascular events like MI, unstable angina and sudden death, as well as a five-fold increased risk for stroke and TIA. Levels of Lp-PLA$_2$ of less than 200 nanograms/mL (ng/mL) are considered low risk, between 200 and 235 ng/mL are intermediate risk, and above 235 ng/mL are considered high risk.

Genetic Markers

Genetic markers are a very active area of interest in many branches of medicine. We have already discussed several diseases of cholesterol metabolism that have been identified to result from genetic defects. There appear to be significant genetic influences on many components of the process of atherosclerosis. By identifying the genetic defects and developing ways to identify patients at risk, genetic testing affords an untapped opportunity to initiate treatment and prevention programs at a very early stage. Genetic testing can also identify which patients are in need for aggressive treatment strategies and, in some cases, also help identify patients in whom there is no need for medications. Genetic testing, unlike standard and advanced lipid testing, which is repeated periodically to assess a change in a patient's CHD risk or response to treatment, needs to be performed only once.

Apolipoprotein E. The gene for apolipoprotein E (Apo E) is found in association with a number of lipid particles, including chylomicrons, VLDLs and HDLs. Just as Apo A does for HDL, and Apo B100 does for LDL, the Apo E apolipoprotein serves to attach its lipid particles to Apo E receptors. An individual's Apo E status is unique and completely under genetic control. Three common types of Apo E apolipoproteins, or isoforms, are made by the Apo E gene: E2, E3 and E4. These are coded for by the corresponding specific chromosomal gene pairs, or alleles. Since each chromosome has two alleles, there are six different combinations, or genotypes, that can result. These are signified by the small-case letter designations; e2/e2, e2/e3, e2/e4, e3/e3, e3/e4 and e4/e4. These genotypes reflect differences in the ability of the Apo E apolipoprotein to attach to Apo E cellular receptors.

There are several important implications to having certain Apo E genotypes. Over 60 percent of the population has an Apo E3 isoform and the Apo e3/e3 genotype. These individuals are usually not at an increased risk for CHD beyond what would be predicted by their other risk factors. The Apo E2 isoform is the least common, occurring in ten to twelve percent of individuals. These individuals have the genotypes Apo e2/e2, Apo e2/e3 and Apo e2/e4. Such patients are prone to markedly elevated triglycerides, usually respond well to treatment with exercise and statin medications to reduce LDL, and also respond well to moderate alcohol consumption to raise HDL. Their lipid abnormalities do not respond well to low-fat diets.

The Apo E4 isoform occurs in 25 percent of individuals, and results in the Apo e3/e4 and Apo e4/e4 genotypes. It is especially associated with a very high risk of CHD due to increased levels of both LDL-C and triglycerides, especially when diets are high in saturated fat. A patient with the Apo E4 isoform needs aggressive treatment and surveillance for CHD. The management of lipid abnormalities in these patients can also be very complex as these individuals also have a very limited ability to reduce LDL with statin medications, although they often respond very well to fat-reduced diets. Apo E4 patients also appear to be at increased risk of developing Alzheimer's disease.

KIF6 Genotype. An increased risk for CHD is also predicted by the kinesin-like protein 6 gene (KIF6). Recall that DNA consists of two strands of amino acids that are linked together in a double-helix conformation, with a sequence of these amino acids of variable length coding for a gene. The pairing of individual amino acids linked to each other is termed a "base pair." Most genes consist of several hundred, up to several thousand, base pairs. The KIF6 gene can become defective through an abnormality in only one base pair of the DNA that constitutes this gene. When the arginine base at position number 719 on the KIF6 gene is lacking, a condition known as 719Arg polymorphism, it predicts an increased risk of CHD anywhere from 30 percent to 55 percent. Such patients are called KIF6 carriers.

The KIF6 gene variant is fairly common, present in up to 60 percent of patients. The defective gene appears to make such patients prone to increased inflammation in the arterial wall, which promotes atherosclerosis. Thus, individuals who are KIF6 positive need aggressive therapies and monitoring for CHD prevention and treatment. The good news is that while these patients have an increased risk of CHD, they also appear to respond exceptionally well to statin medications in reducing LDL-C and CHD risk.

9p21 Genotype. Sequence variants within the 9p21 locus of chromosome nine have also been shown to identify patients at both a higher risk for CHD overall and a higher risk of CHD at an early age. Such patients are known as carriers of the 9p21 genotype. They have twice the risk of having an MI at a young age (men before the age of 50 and women before the age of 60), than non-carriers. Carriers of the 9p21 genotype also have a 30 percent higher risk of CHD at any age and up to a 50 percent higher risk of aortic aneurysm. This risk appears to be in addition to traditional risk factors and family history. By identifying carriers of 9p21, it is possible to initiate treatment strategies at an early stage to prevent CHD.

Chapter 8
The Clinical Aspects of Coronary Heart Disease:
Do You Have It, and If So, When Do You
Call in the Plumber?

WE HAVE DISCUSSED in detail the mechanisms by which atherosclerosis occur, and that one of the most serious consequences of atherosclerosis is the development of CHD (coronary heart disease). In this
chapter we will expand on our knowledge of the clinical aspects of CHD.
We will tie in the principles that we have already discussed with respect to
what happens in CHD at the molecular, microscopic and bird's-eye levels
to what is happening in the individual as a whole. We will discuss the common symptoms, signs and methods for diagnosis. Despite our emphasis on
managing CHD through prevention, nearly two million Americans a year
undergo interventional and surgical therapies for CHD. There remains a
significant debate as to whether these invasive therapies are overused or
inappropriately used. This chapter will provide an overview of what these
therapies are, and in whom the scientific data indicates they should be utilized, and in whom less invasive treatments may work as well.

Symptoms and Signs
The most common symptom of CHD is chest pain. In Chapter two we
introduced the concept that an imbalance in the proportion of blood supply

relative to the demands of the heart causes the condition of ischemia. Since the heart muscle or myocardium needs a robust blood supply to provide it with the energy to work continuously and without interruption, any deprivation in blood supply will affect the function of the myocardium.

> **Illumination:** On average the heart contracts 60 times a minute, 60 minutes per hour, for 24 hours per day without interruption. For the average individual with a life-expectancy in the U.S. currently at just about 80 years of age, this works out to around 2.5 billion heart beats in an average lifetime! No other organ in the body is required to expend this much effort.

When the deprivation in blood supply is temporary and reversible, the resultant ischemia often causes the perception of chest pain, termed angina. This occurs because the reduced oxygen to the myocardium causes stress on the muscle cells of the left ventricle. This is analogous to the lactic acid "burn" that occurs when you stress your skeletal muscles during a vigorous workout. If the blood flow to the tissue is improved, myocardial ischemia can be reversed, and the chest pain improves. If the blood flow remains impaired, the ischemia can progress to infarction, meaning that the tissue has been deprived of oxygen-rich blood for enough time to be permanently damaged. A myocardial infarction is also known as an MI, or commonly, a heart attack.

As we have discussed previously, while an MI is almost always associated with some degree of arterial plaque, in most instances it is not the obstruction from the plaque that causes the MI. Instead, most MIs are caused by rupture of the fibrous capsule that overlies the plaque, which leads to the development of a blood clot inside the coronary artery. An MI can occur with minimal narrowing of the coronary artery caused by plaque.

Not all chest pains are indicative of angina or an MI. In fact, about 80 percent of instances of chest pain for which people seek medical attention have nothing to do with the heart. Therefore, evaluating the characteristics of the chest pains, as well as performing more specific testing to determine the cause, is always necessary. Chest pain is more likely to be caused by the heart if it occurs with physical stress. Other features of chest pain that suggest a relationship to the heart are if it spreads to the left arm or the neck, back, throat or jaw. Often numbness or loss of feeling in the arms, shoulders or wrists may also occur. The character of angina in women is very different than it is in men. In fact, less than half of all women having a heart attack report chest pain as a prominent symptom. Instead, shortness of breath, nausea, indigestion and shoulder pain are more common symptoms. This is one reason why many women with CHD are often misdiagnosed.

When chest pains caused by angina occur in a predictable pattern, most often with activity in a regular pattern over a period of time, it is termed stable angina and is usually associated with high-grade but stable narrowing of the coronary arteries. Angina becomes unstable when it exhibits a pattern of change in its intensity, character, or frequency. Angina occurring with minimal or no activity is also considered unstable. Like stable angina, unstable angina may also indicate a very severe narrowing of the coronary artery. However, the unstable pattern is often caused by either a rapidly increasing level of plaque, or more commonly, a plaque that is nearing the stage of rupture. Unstable angina may precede myocardial infarction and requires urgent medical attention.

The same type of chest pain occurring in angina can also occur during an MI. Other symptoms of an MI can include nausea, dizziness, excessive perspiration and shortness of breath. When an MI occurs, in many instances the damage to the heart muscle is permanent and irreversible. A large single heart attack or many smaller heart attacks can cause weakening of the heart muscle, resulting in congestive heart failure (CHF) or, if permanent damage exists, a condition called cardiomyopathy. Either temporary lack of oxygen to the heart muscle or scar tissue from permanent heart muscle damage can lead to arrhythmias of the heart, which if severe enough can be fatal.

When CHF or arrhythmias develop as a result of either angina or MI, additional symptoms may occur. These include swelling in the legs, also called edema. Breathing difficulties can occur either with exertion or at rest, particularly requiring elevation of the head to relieve symptoms. Dizziness, fainting spells and palpitations may also occur.

Diagnostic Testing for CHD

The diagnosis of CHD depends on an accurate history, a thorough physical examination and an assessment of CHD risk factors, including blood examinations and noninvasive screening exams such as electrocardiograms (ECGs). If an adequate suspicion of CHD exists, more sophisticated testing to accurately determine the extent, location, severity and, most important, the proper treatment of CHD and other associated conditions is then indicated.

The area of greatest interest in advanced cardiovascular testing for CHD is the accurate diagnosis of coronary artery atherosclerotic plaque. Most noninvasive tests to detect coronary plaque rely upon the principle that a level of plaque that causes more than 50–75 percent of the interior of the artery to be narrowed will result in ischemia. This guideline was established from the results of both animal and human studies that indicated that the heart could continue to get sufficient blood supply under most circumstances unless the level of plaque exceeded the 50–75 percent threshold of narrowing of the arterial opening. Thus, all forms of stress testing are designed with this in mind. The diagnosis of angina causing chest pain is typically not confirmed unless there is evidence that this level of obstruction exists. Coronary interventions such as angioplasty and stenting are rarely performed unless this level of obstruction is detected.

Recall from our previous discussion that most heart attacks, and in some cases angina, sudden death and serious arrhythmias occur with much less than 50–75 percent coronary artery obstruction. Therein lies one of the major problems with sophisticated cardiovascular testing for CHD. It is designed to detect a level of plaque that is often more severe than the kind that most often causes heart attacks. Therefore, for an aggressive strategy of prevention and reversal, any amount of plaque should be considered potentially serious and worthy of treatment.

In addition to the evaluation of coronary plaque, the assessment of other aspects of the heart may also be useful. The measurement of the vigor of the left ventricle, also known as left ventricular function, is very important. This can provide evidence of previous damage to the myocardium and the presence of scar tissue. The overall vigor of the heart is expressed by a number called the ejection fraction (EF). This number measures what percentage of the blood inside the left ventricle is pumped out with each heartbeat. An EF above 55 percent is considered normal. An EF below 30 percent is considered severely reduced.

> **Illumination:** The single-most important predictor of prognosis, life expectancy and quality of life in patients with CHD is their EF measurement.

Heart testing also helps to identify disturbances and abnormalities in a number of other areas. Malfunction of the heart valves may often accompany or be caused by an MI or ischemia. The mitral valve, which connects the left atrium to the left ventricle, appears to be especially sensitive to this. Evaluation of the heart valves may guide specific treatments to relieve valve malfunction. Abnormal heart rhythms such as atrial fibrillation or ventricular arrhythmias may also occur in patients with CHD or MI. When identified, treatment may be directed at improving or controlling the heart rhythm through medications, pacemakers or defibrillators. In some instances, very sophisticated evaluation of the pressures, efficiency and function of the various chambers of the heart may be necessary to diagnose either complex problems, or problems that are at a very early stage.

Electrocardiogram. The electrocardiogram (also known as ECG or EKG) is a recording of the electrical activity of the heart. It can be done at the bedside using a small, portable recording instrument that is available in most medical clinics and offices. It is a fairly crude test in the overall armamentarium of heart testing. This is because the reading may be normal in patients with very severe heart disease, and it may be abnormal in patients with very minimal or no heart abnormalities. It is generally considered a screening examination, which supplements the medical history, physical examination and an assessment of cardiac risk factors. The ECG is most useful in someone who has active chest pain, because the recording will often show very typical abnormalities that can lead to an early diagnosis of MI or angina.

Echocardiography. Similar to sonar, echocardiography uses reflected high-frequency sound waves to create electronic images of the heart. A small hand-held sound probe is placed over the front of the chest, and the signals are converted into an electronic image of the beating heart. The instrument is the same instrument used to perform an ultrasound in a pregnant woman to visualize the fetus.

In addition to being entirely noninvasive and completely safe, it is the least expensive of all imaging techniques. It utilizes no radiation and is the only imaging test that provides real-time images, meaning the pictures reflect what is actually occurring at that moment. The echocardiogram is completely portable, making it much more accessible than other advanced cardiac imaging modalities. It is often performed at the patient's bedside in the hospital, and in many physician offices and outpatient diagnostic centers.

This same basic instrument is used to perform other forms of heart and blood vessel ultrasound imaging as well. Ultrasound can provide high-resolution images of the carotid arteries. Recall that carotid imaging that measures carotid intimal medial thickness (cIMT) is a valuable screening tool for CHD. In some cases ultrasound of the heart is performed using an instrument that is easily swallowed and placed in the esophagus during the examination. This technique is called transesophageal echo (TEE), and is an excellent way to provide high-quality ultrasound pictures of the heart from the esophagus. The advantage of the TEE is that the pictures obtained from the esophagus provide a look from behind the heart, and they are often clearer and more accurate than the standard echocardiogram. TEE can also show structures within the heart as well as the aorta that cannot be seen in a conventional echocardiogram.

When echocardiography is combined with Doppler signals, the resulting Doppler echocardiogram provides information about structure, physiology and blood flow within the heart. While Doppler echocardiography does not provide sufficient detail to visualize most coronary arteries, this examination is now considered the gold standard by which to assess heart valve defects, congenital heart diseases and the size and vigor of the left ventricle. In addition, it is the only noninvasive way to measure blood pressures and other sophisticated measurements of blood flow within the internal heart chambers.

Most recently, several new echocardiographic techniques have emerged. Three-dimensional echocardiography (3-D echo) permits views of the heart from almost any angle, revealing previously difficult-to-image structures. More accurate and realistic assessments of heart function, valve function and internal disorders are thereby possible using 3-D echo. It has been particularly valuable in assisting in the surgical evaluations of heart valve disorders as well as the efficiency of left ventricular contraction.

The intracoronary ultrasound (ICUS) and the Doppler flow probe are two new echocardiographic techniques that use a miniaturized ultrasound and Doppler transmitter that are placed on the tip of a small instrument called a catheter. The ICUS provides previously unavailable 360-degree, cross-sectional ultrasound pictures of the coronary arteries from within the blood vessel. Unlike the coronary angiogram that is obtained during a cardiac catheterization procedure, ICUS not only provides a picture of the walls of the artery, it can also directly visualize plaque and the various layers of the arterial wall in detail. The Doppler flow probe can measure pressures within the coronary arteries and can provide more information about the severity and the physics of blood flow through a blockage. Both ICUS and the Doppler flow probe can detect very early levels of plaque. However, both ICUS and Doppler flow probes require a catheter probe inserted directly into an artery. Thus, both are performed during a catheterization and are highly invasive. However, use of these techniques during catheterization has been shown to help better guide the interventional treatment of coronary plaque.

Cardiac Stress Testing. In a stress test, the heart muscle is made to work harder than when it is in a resting state. It is thus caused to consume more oxygen. If there is an imbalance in oxygen supply and demand, it should be reflected in tests that measure the function of the heart muscle. The most common type of stress test involves a recording of the ECG before, during and after a supervised, gradually increasing level of exercise. The exercise is usually done on a treadmill or stationary bicycle while the patient is attached to an ECG monitor. In patients unable to exercise, stress on the heart can be simulated through the use of chemical agents.

With the proper precautions and safety equipment, these examinations are exceedingly safe, with a major complication rate of less than one in 100,000. The accuracy of the test is affected by a variety of issues, including the level of effort of the patient, the likelihood of discovering CHD and the accuracy of the ECG signals, to name only a few. On average, the standard stress test provides accurate readings between 70 percent and 90 percent of the time. Accuracy can be improved when stress testing is combined with echocardiography or cardiac nuclear imaging called scintigraphy.

Cardiac Nuclear Scintigraphy. Nuclear scintigraphy of the heart yields pictures of the heart using intravenously injected radioactive isotopes. Nuclear cardiac imaging is usually performed in conjunction with stress testing as a non-invasive method to identify CHD. Small amounts of radioactive isotopes bound to inert chemicals that target heart muscle are injected into the bloodstream through an arm vein. As these chemicals circulate through the heart, a camera positioned in front of the chest detects the emitted radioactive signals and thus provides information about blood flow to various regions of the heart. Impaired blood flow is a sign of either previous heart damage or ischemia due to a coronary blockage that may be jeopardizing heart muscle that is at risk for future damage.

In the last few years, new computer-based analysis techniques, called SPECT (Single-Photon Emission Computerized Tomography) imaging, and better isotopes, like technetium-99, have improved accuracy rates of nuclear scintigraphy to detect obstructive CHD to better than 95 percent. However, the testing still requires substantial radiation exposure and will still require an angiogram to specifically identify the location and severity of the plaque, and also to treat cholesterol plaque causing a coronary blockage.

Computerized Axial Tomography (CAT). We have previously discussed the role of cardiac CAT scan imaging as a means for CHD screening by the noninvasive detection and measurement of the amount of calcium in the coronary artery. This method, known as CAT scan calcium scoring (CCS), has been shown to demonstrate a correspondence between CCS and the total amount of plaque. The CCS has also been shown to somewhat correlate with the likelihood of developing CHD. However, the amount of calcium in a specific blockage does not correlate with the severity of blockage. Therefore, while calcium scoring may be a good screening tool, it cannot accurately determine the severity of blockage, and thus cannot identify which patients would likely benefit from specific treatments such as medications, angioplasty, stenting or bypass surgery.

The newest generation of CAT scanners, called "multislice" scanners, can obtain x-rays at very high speed and in very thin virtual layers, revealing "slices" of the heart. The standard 64-slice and the newest 256-slice scanners yield high-resolution images of the exterior and interior heart structures, such as the chambers and valves, as well as the coronary arteries, which can be displayed in realistic and anatomically correct fashion. Recent studies indicate that multislice cardiac CAT scan examinations have accuracy rates for detecting CHD exceeding 90 percent. However, CAT scans also have drawbacks that include high radiation exposure (in some cases two to five times as much as in a cardiac catheterization), the need to use iodine dye, and they provide only limited physiologic or blood flow information.

Cardiac Catheterization. The gold standard in cardiac imaging and diagnosis continues to be cardiac catheterization and angiography. The catheterization is done by making a needle puncture in a large artery beneath the skin surface and passing a small flexible tube (catheter) into the heart. The angiogram images of the blood vessels result from the x-rays taken while iodine dye is injected through the catheter into the coronary artery. A catheterization is the only way by which angioplasty and stent procedures can be performed inside a coronary artery.

> **Alert!** There are an estimated four million coronary angiograms performed annually in the world. Over one-half, or two million, are done just in North America.

Despite its widespread use and reliance, angiography still has significant limitations. It provides images that are only a silhouette of the border between the artery and its interior wall and provides little physiologic information. While exceedingly safe, with an incidence of major complications like stroke, heart attack and death in about one in 2,000 cases, it still requires instruments and tubes to be inserted into the blood vessels and chambers of the heart. It requires the use of iodine dye, which can rarely cause allergic reactions as well as kidney failure. Catheterization also requires radiation exposure and is the most costly of the cardiac diagnostic techniques. Many of the new imaging techniques offer the significant advantage of being potentially less costly and non-invasive, causing little to no discomfort or risk associated with the testing. However, the non-invasive techniques do not permit the performance of a coronary interventional procedure such as angioplasty or a stent.

Next-Generation Imaging: MRI and PET Scans. Advanced methods of cardiac imaging are increasingly being used as they become more available, affordable and accurate. One of the major reasons for this is that these imaging methods significantly reduce or eliminate radiation exposure. As noted above, all types of current, commonly used cardiac imaging, except Doppler ultrasound and echocardiography, require radiation. This is true for nuclear scintigraphy, CAT scans and cardiac catheterization.

> **Alert!** The biological effect of ionizing radiation is typically quantified by dose measurements in units of milli-sieverts (mSv). In the United States, the level of annual radiation exposure in the general public has doubled since 1980, from 3.2 mSv to 6.2 mSv in 2010. Medical imaging now accounts for 25 percent of the total annual radiation exposure in the general population. Furthermore, cardiac imaging accounts for 22 percent of all of the medical imaging-related radiation exposure.

Magnetic resonance imaging (MRI) maps radio signals absorbed and emitted by hydrogen nuclei in biological tissue when exposed to a powerful magnetic field. Hydrogen is naturally abundant in the body in the form of water, H_2O. Cardiac MRI offers many advantages for cardiac diagnosis. It is non-invasive and uses neither radiation nor iodine dye. It can accurately visualize many structures, including cardiac chambers, valves and coronary arteries. For the diagnosis of CHD, MRI can provide both structural and blood flow physiologic information, theoretically offering an advantage over both SPECT imaging and cardiac catheterization. It may be the best test to accurately measure heart chamber sizes and evaluate internal heart disorders. Limitations in resolution still exist and access to equipment is fairly limited, so MRI is not yet recommended for routine detection of CHD. Furthermore, MRI cannot be performed in patients with most types of pacemakers or with defibrillators or those who have metallic fragments in or near vital structures.

Cardiac positron-emission tomography (PET) is more readily available than cardiac MRI. PET appears to be the most likely imaging technique to overtake cardiac SPECT nuclear imaging as the preferred method for the non-invasive diagnosis of CHD. PET causes radiation exposure of only 25 percent of that from traditional SPECT nuclear scintigraphy. PET has accuracy rates to detect CHD above 90 percent, similar to SPECT nuclear scintigraphy, and like SPECT, is also non-invasive and extremely safe. PET has the additional capability to not only diagnose blockages in coronary arteries, but can also quantify the severity of blood flow reduction, something traditional SPECT imaging cannot do.

Interventional Treatments for CHD

The focus of this book is on prevention and reversal of CHD. However, there are millions of people who have CHD that is so extensive, lifestyle limiting, or life threatening that they are in need of treatments that restore blood supply to the heart. However, with over two million people worldwide having such treatments, over one-half of them in the United States, there is a significant debate about the appropriateness of these procedures in all patients to whom they are recommended. An overview of these treatments, as well as which types of patients are likely to derive benefit, is presented in this section.

Angioplasty. Percutaneous coronary intervention (PCI) is the general term applied to all types of coronary angioplasty procedures. The PCI procedure extends the diagnostic capabilities of a coronary angiogram performed during a cardiac catheterization to the capability to perform a therapeutic intervention. The physician makes the catheter entry into the arterial system of the body via a needle puncture into an artery in either the leg (femoral artery) or arm (radial artery) without performing an incision, hence the name percutaneous, which means "through the skin surface."

These procedures are used to treat blockages in the coronary arteries caused by varying degrees of plaque and/or thrombosis. In general, only blockages causing more than a 70 percent area of narrowing inside the artery will benefit from PCI. The relief of such partial blockages can improve blood flow to the heart, and the procedure is therefore used to treat both stable and unstable angina. PCI is also used during a heart attack, when the coronary artery is usually completely blocked, to restore blood flow and prevent further heart damage. In the setting of an acute MI, PCI can be immediately lifesaving.

When the procedure was first developed in 1977, it involved only the performance of simple angioplasty, or PTCA (percutaneous transluminal coronary angioplasty), in which a catheter with a deflated balloon on its tip was threaded inside the coronary artery, and the balloon was inflated at the site of blockage to widen the artery. As the range of procedures performed inside the coronary artery has increased, the name of the procedure has changed to percutaneous coronary intervention (PCI).

The most common type of PCI procedure currently performed is the implantation of a stent inside the coronary artery. More than one million stents are implanted annually in the United States to treat coronary artery blockages, making stents the most commonly used medical device. The stent procedure offers the additional advantage over PTCA in that the risk of recurrence of the blockage (restenosis) is significantly reduced. In traditional PTCA, the risk of restenosis was as high as 50 percent within six months. With a stent, the risk of restenosis is about 10 percent.

In a stent procedure, a small flexible tube made of stainless steel wire mesh, the stent, is inserted affixed to the tip of a catheter and wrapped over a deflated balloon. The catheter is threaded to the location of the blockage, and the balloon is inflated. This causes the stent to be "deployed" at the site of blockage. With the application of sufficient pressure from the inflated balloon, the stent is expanded and made to stick into the wall of the interior surface of the artery. The interior of the artery is expanded and the plaque is pushed aside by the stent. The re-growth of plaque and the collapse of the artery are inhibited by the scaffolding properties of the metal stent that tethers the artery open.

Recently, types of stents that are coated with medications that inhibit growth of plaque and scar tissue have been developed. With the gradual release of these medications that seep into the arterial wall, the body's inflammatory and immune response is suppressed, delaying the growth of endothelial cells over the surface of the stent. These stents are called drug-coated or drug-eluting stents (DES), to distinguish them from the traditional bare-metal stent. The DES stents have been shown to further reduce the risk of restenosis. However, since the growth of endothelial cells over the metal struts of the stent is delayed, the metal of the DES is exposed to blood for a longer period of time compared to bare-metal stents. Therefore, some of these stents have a higher risk of blood clots developing within them for up to one year after implantation. This complication carries a high risk of causing an MI and even death. Patients with DES implants are therefore counseled to remain on potent antiplatelet medications without interruption for a minimum of one year after stent placement.

Other forms of PCI include atherectomy, in which a catheter with a rotating blade is inserted into the coronary artery to cut away and extract plaque from the artery. Laser angioplasty is yet another method, in which a laser beam is focused onto an area of plaque through a catheter to dissolve the plaque. In situations where there is also a large amount of blood clot inside the artery, the PCI can include aspiration thrombectomy, in which the blood clot is sucked out of the artery with a vacuum catheter, usually followed by implantation of a stent.

All forms of PCI carry risks associated with the procedure. The procedure is usually performed under local anesthesia with mild sedation. Minor bleeding from the insertion point in the groin or arm is common, in part due to the use of antiplatelet-clotting drugs. As is the case in a diagnostic catheterization, allergic reactions and kidney failure due to the iodine dye can rarely occur. The most serious risks are death, MI and stroke. An MI after PCI will occur in 0.3 percent of cases, and a stroke in 0.1 percent. The need for an emergency bypass during a PCI is very rare. Less than two percent of patients die during a PCI, almost all being those who are undergoing PCI for the treatment of an acute MI.

A number of studies have compared PCI to both medications and bypass surgery, the other forms of therapy for CHD. PCI is an effective therapy for patients with angina. It is especially useful in patients with angina who do not respond to medications. However, for patients with stable CHD, who are not in the midst of an acute MI, there is little evidence to support the premise that PCI is superior to medications in reducing the future risk of MI or death.

A large, randomized controlled trial involving over 2,000 patients called the COURAGE trial (Clinical Outcomes Utilizing Revascularization and Aggressive Drug Evaluation) was published in 2007. This trial concluded that treating patients for stable coronary artery disease with PCI did not reduce the risk of death, myocardial infarction or other major cardiovascular events when added to standard medical treatment. The results of this trial confirmed findings of multiple other previous trials comparing PCI to medications.

The value of PCI in rescuing someone having a heart attack (by immediately alleviating an obstruction) is undisputed. Patients who have significant angina symptoms not responding to medications will likely benefit from stents. However, based upon the substantial scientific data, unless you are in one of these two groups, you should seriously question a recommendation that you have a stent inserted.

> **Illumination:** One touchy issue among interventional cardiologists is that they must battle through their potential conflict of interest in recommending a stent. If the interventional cardiologist derives benefit from placing a stent, economic or otherwise, all else being equal, he or she will generally prefer to recommend a stent. This has tongue-in-cheek been termed the "oculo-plastic reflex," meaning that the "ocular" effect of simply seeing any blockage in the coronary artery reflexively causes the interventional cardiologist to want to remodel or "plasty" the blockage. This only serves to add fuel to the fire in the debate of the appropriateness of stents and angioplasty in managing stable CHD.

Given the ongoing controversy about overutilization of stents, in a non-emergency situation you should consider getting a second opinion from a non-interventional cardiologist before agreeing to have a stent. Make sure you understand why a stent is recommended. Does your stress test or any of the other findings indicate that you are at imminent risk for significant heart damage if a blockage is not relieved by a stent?

In the treatment of a coronary blockage that results in a 70 percent or more area of narrowing within the artery, in a patient who has confirmed angina despite good medical therapy, or is believed to be at significant risk of heart damage, the performance of PCI is generally without controversy. However, if you have a blockage that is causing between 40 percent and 70 percent narrowing of the interior of the artery, the benefits of PCI are much less clear. In this case, it is advisable for the interventional cardiologist to use a Doppler flow probe to measure your fractional flow reserve (FFR). This technique can be performed at the same time as the cardiac catheterization and will provide information about the physics of the blood flow through the area of blockage. If the blockage is serious enough to substantially impair blood flow, the FFR will be abnormal, below a value of 75–80 percent. The FFR provides independent and objective confirmation of the severity of a coronary blockage. Recent clinical trials have shown that when the FFR was used to help decide if a stent was needed, nearly two-thirds of patients avoided getting stents, without any adverse consequences.

Coronary Artery Bypass Surgery. Open heart surgery in which blood flow is re-routed around blocked coronary arteries is the most invasive and drastic procedure to treat CHD. The medical terms for this procedure are coronary artery bypass graft (CABG) or aorto-coronary bypass (ACBP) surgery. The first CABG operations were performed in 1960, and the procedure continues to be an excellent way to treat CHD. However, primarily because of an increased reliance in the use of PCI, the number of CABG procedures has seen a steady decline since its peak in the U.S. in the late 1990s. Between 1996 and 2003, there were 25 percent fewer CABG procedures. A recent study confirmed that the trend has continued, with a further 38 percent decline between 2001 and 2008. In 2010, only about 400,000 CABG procedures were performed in the U.S. Over one-half of all CABG procedures in the world are performed in the U.S.

CABG is now typically reserved for selected patients. Those patients who have either failed PCI or those who have blockages that are too numerous or extensive for PCI to correct are candidates for CABG. Also patients who have blockages that are in vital spots, such as the left main coronary artery where PCI would be too risky, or for patients who have ongoing and severe angina despite good medical therapy and are no longer candidates for PCI by virtue of the progressive and diffuse nature of their blockages should be offered CABG. Certain patients with specific medical conditions, who have severe CHD, have also been shown to have better outcomes with CABG than PCI. Among such patients are diabetics and those with poor left ventricular function.

As a result of a greater level of patient selection in candidates for CABG and the more frequent use of PCI, whereas at one time a typical CABG procedure implanted one or two bypasses, now the typical procedure performed is three or four bypasses. While the number of bypasses performed adds little additional risk to the procedure itself, it indicates that patients undergoing CABG procedures today are overall less healthy and have more extensive CHD than in previous years. Still, CABG is a highly effective way to relieve angina, reduce the risk of future heart attacks, and improve longevity and the quality of life in selected patients with CHD.

In a CABG operation, a detour is constructed around one or more blockages in coronary arteries using grafts or conduits from veins or arteries extracted from other parts of the patient's body. It is always preferable to have one of the bypasses using the left internal mammary artery (LIMA) as the longevity of this bypass far exceeds that for vein bypasses. The bypass of blood around the blocked artery restores blood flow to the areas of the heart that were deprived of blood. In most instances, the surgery requires an incision through the breastbone and requires the heart to be temporarily stopped for the surgeon to implant the bypasses.

Before the CABG procedure, the surgeon reviews the cardiac catheterization angiogram to determine which coronary arteries need to be bypassed. Any blockage that exceeds a level of 50 percent obstruction is typically treated, unless the artery receiving the bypass is either too small or so extensively affected by plaque that is unsuitable to sew in a bypass graft.

During the operation, the patient is put under general anesthesia and the bypass conduits are harvested from either leg veins or arteries, typically from the arm or chest wall. Through the opening in the breastbone, the surgeon retracts the rib cage and exposes the heart. The blood flow within the heart is re-routed to a heart-lung machine, also known as a cardiopulmonary bypass pump. This machine keeps blood circulating to the vital organs of the body, including the brain, kidneys and legs while the heart is stopped. To sew in the bypasses, the surgeon must stop the heart using an ice cold solution of chemicals called cardioplegia. It usually takes between 30–90 minutes to complete the bypasses, at which time the heart is warmed back up, and re-started with a small electric shock administered directly to its surface. Once the heart is beating again, the heart-lung machine is turned off and the blood is allowed to re-enter the heart to be re-circulated to the rest of the body. The layers of tissue in the chest are sewn back together, and wires are used to reattach the breastbone, completing the operation.

Several alternatives to the full CABG procedure have been developed to reduce the risk of complications associated with a prolonged period of time that the heart is stopped and to reduce the pain and complications associated with an incision in the breastbone. One of these is off-pump CABG, in which the surgeon sews in the bypasses on the beating heart, without the need for re-routing blood through the heart-lung machine. A second such procedure is minimally invasive CABG, in which a very small 2–4 inch incision in the chest wall is used, instead of cutting going through the entire breastbone. Both techniques have shown reduced complications, but can be applied only in selected patients. Such patients are those who need only a limited number of bypasses and do not have other complicating medical conditions.

As is the case for PCI, the effectiveness, complications and indications for CABG have been extensively studied in a number of clinical trials. Several large recent trials have compared CABG with PCI. The SYNTAX trial (Synergy Between PCI with Taxus and Cardiac Surgery) was a randomized controlled trial conducted on 1,800 patients who had multiple diseased coronary arteries completed in 2010, and compared CABG versus PCI using drug-eluting stents (DES). The study found that rates of major adverse cardiac events at 12 months were significantly higher in the DES group (17.8 percent versus 12.4 percent for CABG patients). This was primarily due to a higher need for repeat interventional procedures in the PCI group. There was no difference between the two groups with regard to recurrent MI or death rates. Higher rates of strokes were seen in the CABG group.

Two large registry trials have shown CABG to be superior to PCI in many respects. The recent 2012 ASCERT trial (ACCF-STS Database Collaboration on the Comparative Effectiveness of Revascularization Strategies) compared 86,000 patients having CABG to 103,000 having PCI between 2004 and 2007. After four years of follow-up, those who had CABG had a 21 percent lower rate of death than PCI patients. A similar study in 17,000 patients conducted in New York in 2006 also found CABG was superior to PCI with DES in multivessel CHD treated with CABG. Patients having CABG had lower rates of death and MI than stent patients. Patients undergoing CABG also had lower rates of needing repeat procedures to treat obstructions. Both the ASCERT trial and New York State registry were criticized for not being randomized controlled trials, and the patients selected for PCI may have been sicker than those selected for CABG. If this were true, then PCI patients would be expected to do less well than CABG patients.

The prognosis following CABG depends on a variety of factors. The risk of death within the first month after CABG is overall two to three percent. Successful grafts typically last eight to 15 years, although it has been found that 90 percent of LIMA bypasses are still open after ten years. About 40 percent of patients have a new blockage within ten years after CABG surgery. Since CABG does not prevent CHD from recurring, lifestyle changes and long term medication therapy are absolutely essential to maintain optimal health of the bypass grafts as well as the native coronary arteries.

In general, CABG improves the chances of survival of patients who are at high risk, though statistically after about five years the difference in survival rate between those who have had surgery and those treated by medical therapy diminishes. A variety of conditions affect the likelihood of a favorable short and long-term outcome after successful CABG. Patients who are younger, have better left ventricular function, stop smoking, control their lipids and other CHD risk factors, and those in general better health tend to have the best outcomes.

CABG is much more invasive than either medical therapy or PCI. It requires hospitalization typically for four to ten days. After release from the hospital, there is typically a two- to six-week period of convalescence, followed by a three- to six-month period of supervised rehabilitation. This should be compared to PCI recovery when one is evaluating the risks and benefits of one procedure versus the other. An elective PCI typically requires no more than an overnight stay in the hospital and no incision or surgical wound.

People undergoing CABG are at risk for the same complications as any surgery, plus some risks more common with or unique to CABG. These include complications related to wound healing and infection of the breastbone as well as at the vein harvest sites in the legs. The bypass grafts can fail due to development of blood clots or progressive re-growth of plaque or reduced blood flow in the bypasses. Kidney failure, paralysis of the diaphragm, a collapsed lung, fluid in the chest cavity, pneumonia, pulmonary embolism, and heart arrhythmias such as atrial fibrillation are not uncommon complications shortly after CABG.

A full blown stroke complicates CABG surgery in approximately five percent of patients. However, a number of recent studies have found a frequent occurrence of disturbances in mental function soon after CABG. In most instances, these changes are subtle and short-lived, although permanent abnormalities in cognitive function have been reported. One recent study using MRI scans of the brain in patients having CABG found 51 percent of patients had some degree of brain damage. This may be caused by small particles of atherosclerotic debris or micro-blood clots that break loose from the arterial walls, clumps of blood cells, and even plastic tubing and air bubbles that are introduced into the circulation during the CABG operation when the heart is handled or tubes are inserted through blood vessel walls and the blood is diverted into the heart-lung machine.

Chapter 9
Atherosclerosis Outside of the Heart:
Frequently Hidden, Not Always Silent and Sometimes Deadly

AS DISCUSSED IN Chapter two, atherosclerosis can affect almost any artery in the body. Outside of the heart, atherosclerotic cardiovascular disease can also be a major cause of pain, suffering, disability, reduced life expectancy and even sudden death. Furthermore, the occurrence of atherosclerosis in arteries outside of the heart invariably means atherosclerosis also exists inside the coronary arteries. In patients with atherosclerotic cardiovascular disease who do not have clinical evidence of CHD (coronary heart disease), they represent a population that is at high risk for the occurrence of the full spectrum of heart problems, including MI and sudden cardiac death.

The type of atherosclerotic disease outside of the heart has unique symptoms, complications, diagnosis and treatment, depending upon the area of the body that is affected. Even though the clinical syndromes of atherosclerosis outside of the heart are quite varied, they share the same causes, risk factors and pathology. In many cases, they share the same core principles of treatment.

In this chapter, we will review in more detail many of the common clinical syndromes of atherosclerosis outside of the heart. The premise of this book is that the occurrence of these syndromes is preventable.

However, the tools for prevention not only rely upon taking the proper dietary, lifestyle and medical interventions, they also require an awareness of potential symptoms, risks of the disease, methods of diagnosis and treatment options.

Cerebrovascular Atherosclerosis

Atherosclerosis affecting the blood vessels leading to and within the brain is known as cerebrovascular disease (CVD). The two major clinical syndromes associated with CVD are stroke, also known as a cerebrovascular accident (CVA), and transient ischemic attack (TIA). The distinction between CVA and TIA is that, while both cause deficits of neurological function, the deficits in a CVA are permanent, whereas they are only temporary, lasting anywhere from seconds to no more than 24 hours in a TIA.

While a CVA is the general term that describes the sudden and permanent loss of brain function, it can occur from many causes. The most common cause of a CVA is the result of inadequate blood flow to a specific area of the brain. This results in ischemia, or reduced oxygen, to the brain tissue, in much the same way as heart muscle can become ischemic. The buildup of atherosclerotic plaque in the small blood vessels of the brain narrows the opening of the arteries resulting in reduced blood flow. In most instances, a small blood clot also forms at the site of plaque, which results in the sudden development of symptoms of brain dysfunction that characterize a CVA. The development of atherosclerotic plaque follows many of the same mechanisms as in the coronary arteries, and involves the same processes of lipid deposition, inflammation, endothelial dysfunction and thrombosis.

Less common causes of a CVA are atherosclerosis in the large blood vessels in the neck that lead to the brain, the carotid arteries. This may reduce blood flow directly to the brain, or pieces of the plaque may break off, or embolize from the carotid artery and migrate to the brain to interrupt the blood supply. It has recently been recognized that plaque from the upper part of the aorta can also be a source of emboli to the brain to result in a stroke. Even less frequent is the occurrence of a thrombo-embolism, in which a blood clot from blood vessels outside of the brain migrates into the brain blood vessels, leading to an interruption in blood supply. The most common source of a thrombo-embolism is often the heart itself, especially in patients with heart arrhythmias like atrial fibrillation. The least common cause of a CVA is brain damage that occurs due to a hemorrhage of blood that directly seeps into the brain tissue. This can occur if there is an injury to the brain or if a blood vessel bursts inside the brain, leaking the blood into the brain tissue.

A TIA can be caused by all of the same processes that cause a CVA with the exception of brain hemorrhage. In a TIA, the natural protective mechanisms of the body prevent permanent damage to the brain from a reduced supply of blood. These mechanisms include the natural clot-dissolving chemicals in the blood, the capacity of arteries to dilate or enlarge to improve blood flow, and the recruitment of accessory or alternate blood vessels to restore blood supply to the affected area.

In a stroke, the neurological deficits that result from the damage to the brain will correspond to the area of the brain controlling those specific functions. The deficits can be varied and multiple. These can include physical disabilities, such as localized weakness in a part of the body, inability to formulate speech, all the way to partial or even complete paralysis. Sensory deficits involving vision, taste, smell and touch can occur. Finally, cognitive deficits involving memory, attention, and alertness can occur. In most instances, symptoms come on very rapidly, and without prompt attention, the damage to the brain can be permanent in as little as four to six hours from the onset of symptoms. If permanent neurological impairment occurs, the resultant disability can be quite severe. Not only is the quality of a stroke victim's life often severely compromised, statistics indicate that up to 20 percent of stroke victims will die within the first year of their stroke.

As is the case for coronary heart disease (CHD), stroke is very common. It is the leading cause of adult disability in the U.S and is the second leading cause of death worldwide, ranking only after CHD. With few exceptions, the risk factors for stroke closely parallel those for CHD as the causative processes are very similar. Hypertension is more common in stroke victims. Men are 25 percent more likely to suffer strokes than women, yet 60 percent of deaths from stroke occur in women. Since women live longer, they are older on average when they have their strokes and thus more often die as a result of a CVA.

Alert! Some risk factors for stroke apply only to women. Pregnancy, childbirth, menopause and the use of hormone replacement therapy, especially when combined with use of cigarettes, all increase the risk of CVA in women.

Multiple studies have confirmed that silent strokes are much more common than previously realized. A recent study found that when analyzed by sophisticated imaging tests such as MRI, only ten percent of patients with confirmed MRI abnormalities actually had a stroke event in their medical history. In a silent stroke, the neurological deficits are more subtle, such as dizziness, a gradual decline in memory or mental faculties and progressive dementia. The syndrome known as "multi-infarct dementia" is now known to be a common cause of dementia in elderly patients and results from multiple silent strokes. Silent strokes appear to result from the same causes as the more typical strokes, but affect the smaller blood vessels and more limited areas of the brain. The implications of this finding are that there needs to be a greater awareness of the risk of silent strokes in the general population and the medical community. Only then can measures to treat stroke risk factors as well as measures to make an earlier diagnosis be instituted.

The diagnosis of a stroke typically involves many techniques, including a specialized neurological physical examination, as well as imaging tests such as CAT scans, MRI scans, carotid imaging and direct imaging of the cerebral arteries through x-rays and angiography. The diagnosis of stroke itself is clinical, with assistance from the imaging techniques. Imaging techniques primarily assist in determining the location, size, type and cause of the stroke. As of yet, there is no commonly used blood test for stroke, though blood tests may be of help in finding out the likely cause of stroke. Blood tests like the $Lp-PLA_2$ examination have been found to be useful in identifying patients who may be at increased risk of stroke.

Treatment. If caught early enough, a typical stroke caused by atherosclerosis and a blood clot may be treated in a hospital with a stroke center using "clot busters" (thrombolysis). However, less than ten percent of patients with a stroke are able to receive these treatments. For the majority of patients, the management of stroke is typically geared towards recovery of function through rehabilitation and prevention of a future event. Prevention of recurrence requires aggressive attention to modifiable risk factors, including smoking cessation, blood pressure management and control of lipids. Medications that thin the blood by blocking the clumping of the platelets which are responsible for most of the blood clots in the artery are effective in stroke prevention. These include aspirin, as well as more potent medications like clopidrogel (Plavix).

If a significant obstruction caused by atherosclerotic plaque in the carotid arteries is identified, patients may benefit from surgery to open a partially blocked carotid artery in the neck. The typical surgical procedure to do this is called a carotid endarterectomy. Recently, less invasive techniques that employ catheters inserted through the small skin incisions, similar to PCI for CHD have also been developed in which patients can be treated with carotid angioplasty or stents. There is a large body of evidence supporting the value of carotid endarterectomy for preventing a second CVA or TIA in patients who have already experienced such an event. However, for the primary prevention of stroke or TIA in patients discovered to have a carotid blockage, but who have never had symptoms of a CVA or TIA, the use of carotid endarterectomy is controversial and not of proven benefit. The use of percutaneous techniques to treat carotid blockages is an area that is currently under very active investigation.

Peripheral Atherosclerosis

Peripheral atherosclerosis is the occurrence of plaque in arteries outside of the heart and brain. The most common location of these plaque occurrences are in the arteries to the legs. This condition is known as peripheral arterial disease (PAD), or as we will refer to it in this book, peripheral vascular disease (PVD). PVD affects an estimated ten million Americans. Despite its prevalence and cardiovascular risk implications, only 25 percent of PVD patients are under treatment.

The risk factors for PVD are the same as they are for CHD and CVA. Further tightening the link between PVD and other sites of atherosclerosis is the finding that patients with PVD have a four- to five-fold higher risk of

CHD and CVA than do patients without PVD. The symptoms of PVD include leg pain, weakness, numbness, or cramping in muscles due to decreased blood flow, a condition known as claudication. Other symptoms include sores, wounds, or ulcers on the legs and feet that heal slowly or not at all. There may be a noticeable change in color (blueness or paleness) or temperature (coolness) when compared to the other limb. There may be diminished hair and nail growth on affected limbs and digits. Persistent and significantly impaired circulation can lead to death of tissues and gangrene.

> **Alert!** One of the most common and underreported symptoms of PVD is erectile dysfunction (ED) in men. ED is especially associated with several risk factors for PVD, including diabetes and smoking. ED occurs in 25 million American men, with 50 percent of all cases caused by PVD, and an even higher proportion in men over the age of 65 years.

In most cases, PVD may be diagnosed through safe, painless and relatively inexpensive, non-invasive testing. A screening examination called the ABI or ankle-brachial index requires only recordings of blood pressures in the arms and legs simultaneously, and will detect most cases of PVD. Since many patients with PVD have no symptoms, this type of examination will frequently identify patients who may have lurking and silent PVD. More sophisticated testing using ultrasound, Doppler, CAT scan angiography, as well as typical direct contrast angiograms, can localize the areas of atherosclerosis, and help to guide optimal treatment methods.

Treatment. The treatment of PVD depends on how it affects the patient. If the patient experiences claudication that is mild, and there is no significant compromise of blood flow to tissues, conservative therapy is often successful. As in all cases of atherosclerosis, treatment of reversible risk factors such as hypertension, diabetes, lipid disorders, cigarette smoking, etc. is crucial. Physical therapy to promote growth of collateral blood vessels which grow slowly around the blocked arteries is of proven value. Anti-platelet medications like aspirin and Plavix, as well as medications that reduce the viscosity of the blood, such as pentoxifylline (Trental) and cilostazol (Pletal) may also be helpful to improve circulation.

After a trial of the best medical treatment as outlined above, if symptoms remain unacceptable, mechanical treatments to restore the circulation to the legs can be offered. These include the percutaneous procedures of angioplasty and stenting. If the atherosclerosis is extensive, then surgical bypass of the blocked arteries using artificial grafts of Gore-Tex or Dacron can be performed, much in the same way as a heart CABG operation. If gangrene has set in, amputation is often a last resort.

Renal Artery Stenosis

One of the most common places for the development of the silent narrowing of blood vessels is in the main arteries leading to the kidneys. These arteries are called the renal arteries and the condition is known as renal artery stenosis (RAS). This condition is the most common cause of what is known as secondary hypertension. Secondary hypertension is blood pressure elevation caused by something other than the typical high blood pressure condition that is caused by generalized arteriosclerosis. The latter is termed primary hypertension, and afflicts about 100 million Americans. Secondary hypertension is relatively uncommon, occurring in about three to four percent of patients with high blood pressure. RAS is believed to afflict two to three million Americans, and when present and not treated appropriately, it can lead to kidney failure and the need for dialysis. Furthermore, the proper treatment of RAS can often result in either elimination, or a significant reduction in blood pressure medications.

RAS can result from one of two processes in the wall of the renal artery. The most common is typical atherosclerosis, of the type seen in all other arteries. The less common variety is called fibromuscular dysplasia (FMD). The latter typically occurs in young women between 30 and 40 years of age. This is caused by an abnormal thickening of the middle, muscular layer of the renal artery that occurs for unknown reasons. FMD is likely genetic, as it affects Caucasian women much more often than men or black or Asian women. The atherosclerotic variety is associated with the same risk factors as other types of atherosclerosis. It is often associated with atherosclerosis in other spots, including CHD, PVD and aortic atherosclerosis.

Since RAS is silent and without overt symptoms, it can only be detected if the diagnosis is suspected and appropriate testing is performed. Any young patient with unexplained hypertension and any older patient with known risk factors for atherosclerosis or known atherosclerosis should undergo screening examinations. Screening exams for RAS are non-invasive imaging studies like Doppler ultrasound, CAT scans and MRI scans of the aorta and renal arteries.

Treatment. The proper treatment of RAS depends upon the severity. In most patients with mild disease and mild to moderate hypertension, the right types of blood pressure medications typically are effective. Blood pressure medications that work by altering kidney hormones, like angiotensin converting enzyme (ACE) inhibitors, angiotensin receptor blockers (ARB) and direct rennin inhibitors (DRI) are usually contraindicated, since they have been found to worsen kidney function when the renal artery stenosis affects both kidneys. Treatment also involves managing risk factors for atherosclerosis. Given the frequent association of RAS with CHD and other types of atherosclerosis, individuals with RAS should always be screened for CHD, PVD and CVD.

When RAS is moderate to severe, with evidence of difficult to control blood pressures, occurrences of congestive heart failure, evidence of kidney malfunction or the FMD type, an invasive approach is typically recommended. In most instances, this involves the same PCI techniques of angioplasty and stent placement that are used to treat CHD. While this approach is generally successful, it is also controversial. The results of a clinical trial of 200 patients was released in September, 2012 that found stenting for RAS modestly improved blood pressure, but had no effect on kidney function. In especially severe cases of RAS, surgical bypass of the renal arteries can be done. If all else fails, the affected kidney can be removed. However, if both kidneys are involved, and removed, the patient is obviously committed to life-long dialysis.

Aortic Atherosclerosis

Atherosclerosis can affect the aorta, the main artery running through the central part of the body in a variety of ways. In most cases, this process is also silent and without symptoms. In a recent study of nearly 600 patients, typical atherosclerosis, with the development of plaque lining the arterial wall of the aorta was present in over 40 percent of patients by the age of 65 years. The majority of these patients had no symptoms, and plaque was found to be severe in nearly eight percent of patients.

Plaque in the aorta can rarely lead to the narrowing of the opening of the aorta. However, this is much less common than in other arteries since the aorta is so large in caliber and much more elastic than other arteries in the body. In most instances, the consequences related to plaque buildup are the migration or dislodgment of pieces of plaque, a condition known as athero-thrombo-embolism. In this condition, the plaque breaks loose from the wall of the aorta, collects a cluster of platelets within the circulation, and the complex of plaque and blood clot migrates or embolizes to other spots in the body, such as the circulation areas leading to the brain, kidneys and legs. This can lead to stroke, reduced blood flow to regions of the legs, gangrene, and death of kidney tissue resulting in kidney failure. In patients with known severe aortic atherosclerosis, a recent study found that up to 33 percent had a clinical event of athero-thrombo-embolism within one year of their diagnosis. In about one-third of these instances, the event was a CVA.

Since aortic atherosclerosis is usually without symptoms, it must be detected by screening methods targeted to patients with typical risk factors for atherosclerosis, or those who have known CHD, PVD, RAS or CVD. These are the typical non-invasive imaging methods we have previously discussed, and include Doppler ultrasound, transesophageal echo (TEE), CAT scans and MRI. Patients with higher levels of vascular inflammation, as evidenced by elevated levels of CRP or Lp-PLA$_2$, appear to be at an especially higher risk.

Another manifestation of aortic atherosclerosis is the development of a weakening of the normally elastic wall of the aorta. The same risk factors that cause plaque build-up also promote the weakening of the aortic wall. This results in a bulge in the weakened segment of the wall, and if this bulge achieves a size of one and one-half times that of the normal aorta, it is termed an aneurysm. An aneurysm can occur in any segment of the aorta. In the upper aorta, it is called a thoracic aortic aneurysm (TAA), and in the lower aorta, it is called an abdominal aortic aneurysm (AAA). Aside from atherosclerosis, there are also less common causes for aortic aneurysms. Conditions like infections in the aorta, trauma and inflammatory and connective tissue diseases of the aorta account for less than five percent of all aortic aneurysms.

As is the case for most types of atherosclerosis outside the heart, aortic aneurysms are also typically silent, and therefore not detected unless there is reason to suspect they are present, or they are found incidentally in the course of evaluating other medical issues. Left untreated, aortic aneurysms can result in several serious and life-threatening problems. An enlarging aneurysm can put pressure on adjacent organs like the stomach, heart, lungs and nerves. If this occurs, symptoms such as abdominal pain, chest pain, back pain, shortness of breath, hoarseness, and numbness may occur.

Once an aneurysm sufficiently enlarges, it is at risk for rupture. Blood clots can form in the aneurysm and migrate to cause an athero-thrombo-embolism. Finally, a tear in the interior lining of the aorta can occur; this is a condition known as dissection. In this case, the tear can lead to rupture of the aorta, or can compromise the blood supply to the heart, brain, kidneys, intestines, and any other blood vessel connected to the aorta. Collectively, these conditions are responsible for the deaths of over 45,000 Americans per year.

The diagnosis of an aortic aneurysm is usually made using the non-invasive screening tests discussed above. These examinations can not only diagnose the aneurysm, they can also precisely determine the size of the aneurysm, as well as if there is an internal blood clot or dissection. An aortic aneurysm is most likely associated with atherosclerosis, and should be suspected in any patient with atherosclerosis in any other part of the body, and especially in patients who are over the age of 50, have hypertension, smoke or who have a strong family history. Genetic tests like genotype 9p21 predict a significantly increased likelihood of aortic aneurysms.

> **Illumination:** For aortic aneurysms, in terms of risk, size matters.
>
> For thoracic aortic aneurysms, the annual risk of rupture according to size is:
>
> > greater than 4 cm. 0.3%
> > greater than 5 cm. 1.7%
> > greater than 6 cm. 3.6%
>
> For abdominal aortic aneurysms, the annual risk of rupture according to size is:
>
> > greater than 5 cm. 5.0%
> > greater than 6 cm. 5.9%
> > greater than 7 cm. 15%

Aortic rupture most commonly results from an AAA, which accounts for 95 percent of all aortic ruptures. Dissections can occur in either an AAA or TAA. Both are life-threatening events and require immediate surgery. Many AAA dissections can be managed without surgery. However, most TAA, especially those in the most upper parts of the aorta need to have immediate surgery. An aortic dissection, even with surgery, carries a very high mortality rate, with between 70–90 percent of patients not surviving.

Treatment. The medical treatment of patients with aortic atherosclerosis and small, stable aneurysms involves control of the typical risk factors, including absolute abstinence from tobacco, and lipid and blood pressure control. In patients with aortic atherosclerosis, but without evidence of aneurysm, anticoagulant medications may be useful. Antiplatelet medications like aspirin and clopidrogel (Plavix) as well as warfarin have been shown to be beneficial in reducing the risk of embolism. However, both types of medications carry substantial risks. No clinical trial evaluating the use of these medications to prevent embolism in patients with advanced aortic atherosclerosis has been conducted, although one is currently being carried out in Australia and Europe. A recent observational study of over 500 patients with severe aortic atherosclerosis showed that use of stain therapy was associated with a 60 percent reduced risk of embolic events. Studies using TEE in patients with aortic atherosclerosis receiving statin therapy have shown significant plaque regression, plaque stabilization, reduced vascular inflammation and a reduced risk of CVA.

Surgical treatment of an aortic aneurysm is generally advised if the patient has symptoms or the aneurysm reaches a size threshold where there is a dramatic rise in the risk of rupture (TAA, greater than 4 cm; AAA, greater than 5 cm). Aneurysms of smaller size should also be treated surgically if the aneurysm is found to be expanding at a rapid rate.

Open surgery carries substantial risks, not only because of the nature and complexity of the operative procedure, but also because such patients often have co-existing CHD or CVD. In an open operation, the dilated part of the aorta is replaced by a synthetic (Dacron or Gore-Tex) patch tube through an incision in the chest or abdominal cavity. In order to do this, the blood supply in the aorta must be interrupted, which can lead to deprivation in blood flow to the brain, heart and spinal column. Patients undergoing open repair of aneurysms are at a much higher risk of MI, CVA and paralysis.

To reduce the surgical risks associated with open repair, in recent years, the endoluminal treatment of abdominal and also thoracic aneurysms has been of considerable interest and study. This is a minimally invasive procedure that does not require cutting through the chest wall or abdomen. Instead, a stent mesh graft is inserted within the diseased segment of aorta through the femoral artery in the leg. The technique is percutaneous, meaning that it can be done through a small skin incision over the femoral artery, and all instruments and grafts are on catheters that are threaded inside the aorta without having to open the aorta or interrupt its blood supply. The technique is still being evaluated in clinical trials, but early results indicate that it is an excellent option for accomplishing a successful aortic aneurysm repair, with a much lower operative risk in selected patients.

PART III
Therapeutic Strategies and Interventions for the Prevention, Treatment and Reversal of Atherosclerosis

Chapter 10
TLC—Part One:
The First Steps to Good Cardiovascular
Health—Eating to Live

THERAPEUTIC LIFESTYLE CHANGES, abbreviated as TLC, are the first interventions that are recommended to prevent, treat and reverse CHD (coronary heart disease). TLC is an integral component of all U.S. national CHD guidelines put forth by the American Heart Association (AHA), American Diabetes Association (ADA) and the National Cholesterol Education Program (NCEP). It is no coincidence that this abbreviation was chosen, as these steps require an investment of effort, desire and motivation that signifies an individual is willing to exhibit behavior that shows another type of TLC, tender loving care, for his or her heart.

When we speak of TLC, we are talking about interventions that favorably modify diet, body weight, physical activity, tobacco consumption and stress management. The purpose of TLC is to institute lifestyle changes that are known to reduce the risks of CHD and CHD risk factors such as diabetes, metabolic syndrome, hypercholesterolemia, obesity and hypertension. These interventions are intended to be introduced before medications, supplements and other treatments that carry potential risks. In this chapter we will review the postulated and proven benefits of various diet regimens and the consumption of heart-healthy foods as components of an overall

TLC program. The next chapter will discuss the other important components of TLC and the cardiovascular benefits of modifying other CHD risk factors.

Overview of Dietary Interventions

A number of diet plans are available that offer the promise of keeping your heart healthy. Many diets are popular because of their commercial support and simplicity, such as those promoted by Weight Watchers and Jenny Craig. Some have become fashionable through well-promoted programs and books, such as the Zone diet and the Abs diet. New diet plans and books remain exceedingly well received. Unfortunately, how well received diets are has nothing to do with how well they reduce the risk of CHD or improve vitality, metabolism or cholesterol. Their popularity is generally linked to the ease and rapidity by which they promote weight loss. However, typically new diets offer no epiphanies. Most of these diets have their basic principles, with minor variations, in one of the main types of dietary programs discussed below.

In general the main dietary programs can be divided into four types: (1) the traditional and widely endorsed low-fat, low-calorie diets such as the TLC, AHA and DASH diets, (2) extremely low-fat, high-carbohydrate, vegetable-focused diets, like the Pritikin, Ornish and Portfolio diets, (3) the high-protein, low-carbohydrate diets, such as the Atkins and South Beach diets, and (4) the balanced and metabolically focused diets, like the Mediterranean diet. In this section, we will provide an overview of the basic principles and merits of these diets.

We discussed what constitutes an unhealthy diet in terms of its effects on blood lipids and CHD in Chapter five. To briefly review, the unhealthy foods that promote clogging of the arteries are: (1) those high in sodium, because of the increased risk of hypertension associated with their consumption, (2) those high in refined sugar and starches, because of the increased risk of diabetes and metabolic syndrome, and (3) those high in saturated fats, trans-fats and dietary cholesterol. Avoidance of these foods is the primary component of most accepted dietary approaches in cardiovascular disease prevention. What differs among the heart-healthy diets is what types of foods replace the prohibited foods and the scientific principles behind these diets.

Traditional Low-Fat Diets

Therapeutic Lifestyle Change (TLC) and American Heart Association (AHA) Diets. Both the TLC and AHA diets are traditional heart-healthy diets endorsed by the National Cholesterol Education Program and closely follow the guidelines of avoidance of the unhealthy foods described above. Their primary goals are to reduce blood cholesterol and avoid obesity. Both diets can promote weight loss in the short-term, although the weight reduction is much more modest than some of the other diets discussed below. Typically, weight loss is no more than five to fifteen pounds after one year of adherence.

In both TLC and AHA diet programs, total fat intake is restricted to no more that 25–35 percent of total calories. In patients with metabolic syndrome or who are at risk for diabetes, carbohydrate intake should also be reduced to no more than 50 percent of total calories. Saturated fat is restricted to less than seven percent of total calories, the equivalent of about 15 grams in a typical 2,000-calorie diet. Trans-fat intake is completely discouraged, and cholesterol intake is limited to less than 300 milligrams a day if cholesterol levels are normal, and less than 200 milligrams per day if blood cholesterol is high. Sodium intake is restricted to less than 2,300 milligrams a day, but if an individual already has hypertension, the optimal sodium intake should be less than 1,500 milligrams daily.

> **Illumination:** As a reference, examples of these daily AHA and TLC nutritional recommendations are noted in the following foods:
> One teaspoon of salt contains 2,300 milligrams of sodium.
> One McDonald's Quarter Pounder with cheese contains 15 grams of saturated fat.
> One egg contains 150–220 milligrams of cholesterol.

In place of saturated fat and trans-fat, both the TLC and AHA diets encourage an increase in monounsaturated and/or polyunsaturated fats as replacement for saturated fats. The preferred monounsaturated fats are the omega-9 variety, the most prevalent of which is oleic acid. This is typically found in olive oil, avocados, nuts, canola oil and peanut oil. The preferred polyunsaturated fats are the omega-6 and omega-3 variety. The omega-6 variety, the most prevalent of which is linoleic acid, is found in many nuts and seeds, as well as vegetable oils, including sunflower, canola, safflower, corn and soybean oils. The healthiest omega-3 types are found in oily fish (especially salmon, tuna and mackerel).

Other positive effects of monounsaturated and polyunsaturated fats occur when these fats replace dietary carbohydrates. Particularly in over-weight or obese individuals and those with metabolic syndrome and diabetes, reducing complex carbohydrate intake (starches) can significantly improve triglyceride and HDL-C levels, as well as improve insulin resistance. Both the TLC and AHA diets promote replacing refined grains with whole grains. A recent study showed such a dietary change improved blood pressure and lipid values and reduced the risk of CHD. Adherence to both the TLC and AHA diets can be expected to reduce LDL-C by ten to fifteen percent.

Specific to the TLC diet are the recommendations for the addition of plant sterols and stanols. Derived mostly from soybean and tall pine tree oils, these are available in a wide variety of foods, such as margarines, cooking oils, and as nutritional supplements called phytosterol. Maximum dietary effects to reduce LDL-C occur at a dose of two grams a day.

The TLC diet also encourages soluble forms of dietary fiber, which can also reduce LDL-C; at a dose of 10–25 grams per day, LDL-C will drop an additional two to three percent. Soluble fiber also promotes digestive health. Common sources of soluble fiber are fruits, vegetables, legumes and grains.

The AHA has promoted a low-fat diet that very closely follows the principles in the TLC diet for years. In previous years the AHA classified their diet plans as either Step I or Step II, distinguished primarily by the degree of saturated fat restriction. Saturated fat restriction remains a core principle of the current AHA diet. However, the current guidelines for the

AHA diet are intended to be more "user-friendly" as they focus more on specific foods, rather than on complex calculations of cholesterol intake and saturated fats as percentages of food components.

Like the TLC diet, the AHA diet is also primarily intended to lower cholesterol. The AHA diet encourages five types of foods: (1) two weekly servings of cold-water oily fish, such as tuna, salmon, mackerel, lake trout, herring or sardines, (2) a variety of dark green, deep orange or yellow fruits and vegetables, such as spinach, carrots, peaches and berries, (3) 25–30 grams a day of fiber from whole grains, fruits, vegetables and legumes, (4) nonfat, low-fat or reduced-fat dairy products, and (5) liquid vegetable oils and soft margarines in place of butter, hard margarine or shortening.

While the traditional TLC and AHA diets can improve blood lipids, the evidence that they reduce CHD risk is limited. The only large trial exclusively evaluating this type of diet was the MRFIT trial. Conducted in the early 1970s in over 300,000 individuals, the study showed a general relationship between blood cholesterol and CHD events. However, even while participants following a low-fat diet showed small improvements in blood lipids, there was no reduction in cardiovascular events with diet intervention alone. In 2006, the Women's Health Initiative, an eight-year study of 49,000 American women between the ages of 50–79 who followed a reduced fat diet came to the same conclusions.

Both the TLC and AHA diets are promoted as public health initiatives as they have sound scientific principles and modest evidence supporting a benefit in blood lipids and weight loss. Most importantly, they are fairly easy to follow with respect to finding the proper types of foods in the grocery aisle and in restaurants. They also are affordable diets, as they require no exotic or expensive foods, meal plans or recipes. However, many proponents of other diet plans have criticized these diets as being contributors to the ongoing epidemic of obesity, metabolic syndrome and diabetes in American society as they are not effective diets in addressing these risk factors.

DASH Diet. Another nationally endorsed diet worthy of mention is the DASH program. The acronym stands for Dietary Approach to Stopping Hypertension. It was developed by the National Heart, Lung, and Blood Institute (NHLBI) in the 1990s in response to the well-established link between poor dietary habits and development of hypertension. It is not a diet designed to lower cholesterol *per se*. However, because it is calorie and fat restrictive and lowers blood pressure, it is considered a heart-healthy diet. Hypertension is a major CHD risk factor as well as a contributor to chronic kidney disease and, like lipid disorders, affects 100 million Americans.

The principles of the DASH diet derive from promoting an increase in nutrients known to lower blood pressure, specifically fiber, protein, potassium, magnesium and calcium. All of these nutrients are consumed by most Americans in much lower amounts than recommended. For example, potassium intake in the DASH diet is targeted to 4,700 milligrams per day, an amount that is more than double what most Americans consume. To consume this amount of potassium, one would need to eat 11 bananas per day.

The DASH diet is rich in fruits, vegetables, legumes, whole grains, lean meat, fish, poultry, nuts and low-fat dairy foods. It is limited in red meats and fatty foods. It is limited in foods and beverages with added sugar and sodium. DASH suggests capping sodium intake at 2,300 milligrams per day initially, and eventually working towards a goal of 1,500 milligrams per day.

The favorable health effects of the DASH diet are documented by scientific studies. A 2005 study found the DASH diet reduced systolic and diastolic blood pressure by three to six mmHg in patients who did not have hypertension. Patients with hypertension had more profound drops in these values, averaging a reduction of 10–15 mmHg. Some of the most robust results of the DASH diet were reported in a 2006 study of 436 subjects. The DASH diet favorably affected lipids, showing an average LDL-C drop of 17 mg/dL, or about 15 percent of baseline levels, and an HDL rise of 4 mg/dL, or about 10 percent of baseline. In this study, parameters of diabetes were also improved, with subjects showing a 30 percent drop in fasting glucose. On average, weight loss with a DASH diet is eight to fifteen pounds within one year, but as in most diets, the majority of people do not sustain the weight loss. Despite the documented benefits in weight, blood pressure, sugar and lipid reductions, the DASH diet has not yet been shown to reduce the risk of CHD events.

The DASH diet is fairly easy to follow, as it is available as an eating plan published by the NHLBI. The plan works through the process of determining individual daily caloric goals, specific for age and activity status. It apportions permitted foods according to allowed daily servings of the various food groups; grains, vegetables, fruits, dairy, etc. The foods are commonly available and relatively inexpensive, but still more costly than the readily available and cheaper processed fatty, salty and sugary foods most Americans consume. Restricting sodium intake at a restaurant may also be a challenge, as sodium is commonly used in the preparation and preservation of commercial foods. The high intake of potassium, magnesium, calcium and protein in a DASH diet can be harmful to patients with chronic kidney disease.

Low-Fat, High-Carbohydrate, Vegetable-Focused Diets

In the late 1970s and 1980s, Drs. Dean Ornish and Nathan Pritikin led a revolution in conventional dietary approaches to heart disease by studying and promoting extremely low-fat, whole food, plant-based diets combined with significant lifestyle interventions. Ornish and Pritikin sought not just to prevent the occurrence or progression of CHD, but took the ambitious step of employing severe fat restriction to try and reverse CHD. At the time, there were no medications that could dramatically lower blood lipid levels, so their programs were designed to achieve this goal through diet, as well as introduce other favorable lifestyle modifications that they believed would counter the development of CHD.

Ornish Plan. This program promotes very selective, but unrestricted, calorie intake. Ornish categorizes foods into five groups, ranging from the least to most healthful. The goal is to achieve a diet where only ten percent of calories come from fat. Most foods in the least healthful category are those high in cholesterol. Thus, nearly all animal products other than egg whites and small quantities of nonfat milk or yogurt are banned. All refined carbohydrates and oils are banned. Very limited amounts of caffeine and alcohol (up to two ounces of each daily) are permitted. The most healthful are foods high in fiber and complex carbohydrates. Most of the Ornish diet plans yield a sodium intake of much less than the 2,300 milligrams, and a potassium intake of much more than the 4,700 milligrams that are recommended in the traditional heart-healthy diets discussed above. A comparison of the selected

nutritional content of the Pritikin/Ornish plans with the AHA/TLC/DASH
diets and a typical American diet is shown in **Table 10.1**.

Table 10.1

A Comparison of the Selected Nutritional Content of Three Diet Plans

	Pritikin/Ornish	AHA/TLC/DASH	"Typical" American Diet
Fat (% calories/day)	10 or less	25-35	35-45
Protein (% calories/day)	10-15	15-20-	10-15
Carbohydrates	75-80	50-55	40-45
Cholesterol (mg/day)	100 or less	300 or less	450-500
Fiber (grams/day)	35 or more	25-30	10-15
Sodium (mg/day)	1,600 or less	2,300 or less	3,500-6,500
Potassium (mg/day)	5,000 or more	4,700 or more	2, 000 or less

How you eat and live is also emphasized in the Ornish plan. Ornish
suggests eating a lot of little meals, because the composition of the diet
increases hunger for most people. Smaller and more frequent meals reduce
the sensation of hunger without a significant increase in calories. The
Ornish plan also emphasizes the importance of calorie expenditure by
mandating the equivalent of at least 30 minutes of moderate exercise per
day. Finally, some form of stress-management, such as meditation, massage,
psychotherapy or yoga is required.

Dean Ornish reported his initial results in a much ballyhooed randomized controlled study called the Lifestyle Heart Trial in 1990. Patients
with preexisting CHD following the Ornish plan had fewer cardiac events
and reduced the degree of blockage in their coronary arteries within just
one year, compared to patients following standard nutrition and lifestyle
recommendations. The original trial was criticized because it had only 28
subjects in the treatment group. In a subsequent paper, Ornish reported
that the benefits were maintained after five years of follow-up in the same
subjects. The CHD benefits of the Ornish plan have also been subsequently
confirmed in other small studies.

Other documented benefits of the Ornish plan have been shown in
clinical trials. Blood pressure and LDL-C levels are reduced on average by
20 percent. The reported weight loss with the Ornish plan has been

variable, ranging from seven to twenty pounds at one year, with a much smaller maintained benefit after five years of follow-up. Blood sugar levels as well as levels of Hemoglobin A1C, a measure of long-term sugar control improve by five to ten percent in diabetics following the Ornish plan.

Pritikin Program. Like the Ornish plan, this is also a low-fat diet, not vegetarian, but largely based on vegetables, grains and fruits. Total fat intake in the diet accounts for only ten percent of calories. Cholesterol intake is limited to 100 mg/day. The diet is low in protein, with very sparse amounts of meat, dairy and fish intake permitted. It is high in complex carbohydrates, which account for 75–80 percent of total daily calories. Caffeine and alcohol intake are restricted to one or fewer beverages per day.

Nathan Pritikin was educated as an engineer, not a physician. He was afflicted with CHD at the age of 42. His plan was thus partly motivated by his own health condition, and Pritikin followed his plan zealously. Pritikin developed cancer and committed suicide at the age of 69. His autopsy showed no signs of persistent coronary blockages. Pritikin termed his program "mankind's original meal plan," because the focus of the diet is unprocessed or minimally processed straight-from-nature foods. The latest version of the Pritikin plan has been slightly modified and updated by Nathan Pritikin's son, Robert.

The current Pritikin plan emphasizes unlimited amounts of fruits, vegetables, legumes and whole grains. Calorie-dense foods are to be avoided. Instead, low-calorie foods that provide a lot of bulk are encouraged. As in Ornish, the idea is to feel full without consuming significant calories. Also like the Ornish plan, the Pritikin plan emphasizes daily exercise, recommending 30–45 minutes of moderate exercise daily.

There is also sound scientific support for the Pritikin program. In several studies published since 1975, it has been documented that it improves blood lipid profiles better than cholesterol-lowering drugs like statins. Many studies show LDL-C levels drop by 25 percent within one month. The program has also been found to lower blood sugar and blood pressure. Data from the Pritikin centers report an average weight loss of 13 pounds among their clients, although in independent studies, short and long-term maintained weight loss is much less. Some studies have found improvements in inflammatory markers like C-reactive protein and oxidative stress, as well as a reduced incidence of breast, colon and prostate cancer.

A five-year follow-up study of 64 men who came to the Pritikin Longevity Center instead of undergoing bypass surgery (which had been recommended by their heart surgeons) found that 80 percent of these patients never needed the surgery after leaving the center. Of those taking drugs for angina pain, 62 percent left the center drug-free. Of course, the study results have limited applicability since the study was neither blinded nor a randomized trial.

There are a number of criticisms applied to both the Ornish and Pritikin plans. One is that they are very rigid and do not allow a lot of food choices for those used to the western diet. Thus, not many people can stay on them for the long term. Also, many people get tired of eating food with such a low fat content. There is also concern about how severely fat is limited in the two diets, as this may lead to deficiencies in fat-soluble vitamins. Both diet plans require the use of vitamin supplements including B_{12} and fat-soluble vitamins.

These diets also go counter to ample data from numerous studies that show that it is the type of fat, rather than the total amount, that is related to cardiovascular health. There is strong evidence in both epidemiological, population-based studies and clinical trials that monounsaturated and poly-unsaturated fats have a protective effect against coronary heart disease. Ornish, in particular, does not distinguish the good fats from the bad fats. Finally, very low-fat, high-carbohydrate diets may paradoxically increase triglyceride and LDL levels, especially in patients who have insulin resis-tance associated with diabetes or metabolic syndrome.

Portfolio Diet. The Portfolio diet is one of the most intensely studied vegetarian diets. It was introduced by Canadian researchers in 2000. It combines many of the components of a TLC diet (with the exception of meats and dairy products), with a high-fiber, vegetable-based diet similar to the ones promoted by Ornish and Pritikin. Multiple studies of patients using this diet have shown that it dramatically lowers blood lipids. It is sometimes termed the "Simian" diet, as it follows a diet that chimpanzees, gorillas, orangutans and gibbons (simians) follow in the wild. It recommends multiple servings of fruits, vegetables and nuts daily, in addition to the standard fat restriction of traditional diets.

The portfolio diet removes the meat and dairy components of the TLC diet. It replaces them with three additional foods: (1) vegetable protein, derived primarily from soy, beans, lentils and chickpeas, (2) viscous fiber, derived from oats, barley, psyllium, legumes, eggplant and okra, and (3) nuts, mostly almonds and walnuts. It also emphasizes the use of plant sterols and stanols as does the TLC diet.

Each of these components provides additional lipid benefits over what would be expected from a TLC low-saturated-fat diet. An increase in dietary vegetable protein reduces cholesterol production in the liver. An increase in viscous fiber promotes the intestinal elimination of cholesterol in bile acids. Nuts like almonds contain healthy monounsaturated fatty acids that reduce LDL-C. Plant stanols and sterols reduce cholesterol absorption. Each of these four components independently has been shown to reduce LDL-C by an additional five percent.

Clinical trials demonstrate that subjects following the Portfolio diet reduce their LDL-C by 15–30 percent from baseline, a significant difference between the ten percent reduction typically seen with an AHA or TLC diet. The best responders in LDL-C have a response equivalent to the average drop in LDL-C with statin medications. The Portfolio diet also has been shown to reduce CRP levels by 30 percent, reduce triglycerides by ten percent and raise HDL-C by five to ten percent. These average blood lipid improvements are as robust as the best results found by Ornish and Pritikin.

However, while the lipid lowering benefits of the portfolio diet are documented, no clinical studies have yet been completed using the Portfolio diet for benefits in the occurrence of CHD or CHD events. The diet has not been shown to induce or maintain significant weight loss, sugar or blood pressure lowering. The diet is also very difficult to follow for most people as it severely restricts all meat and dairy products.

Low-Carbohydrate, High-Protein Diets

The Atkins and South Beach programs are two popular dietary approaches that are founded on the principle that a low-carbohydrate and high-protein intake is beneficial for blood lipids, weight reduction, metabolism and reduction in CHD risk. Originally published in 1972, *Dr. Atkins' Diet Revolution* was indeed a revolution from the prevailing conventional wisdom that a low-fat diet was the only way to prevent and treat CHD.

Atkins Diet. The basic principle of the Atkins diet is that since carbohydrates are the primary fuel for the body, by restricting carbohydrate intake, the body must turn to its alternative or secondary fuel source: stored fat. Thus, carbohydrate restriction results in a reduction in stored fat and weight loss.

Carbohydrates are the primary form in which the body ingests sugar. Nearly all forms of ingested sugar are converted to the primary sugar that is used by the cells of the body, glucose. When carbohydrate intake is restricted, glucose levels drop. This induces a reduction in the hormone insulin, which we know from our previous discussion is released by the pancreas in response to insulin. The drop in insulin levels promotes the release of fatty acids from the body's fat stores, a process known as lipolysis. The released fatty acids are converted to small carbon fragments called ketones. The presence of ketones in the bloodstream is a condition known as ketosis, and is a sign that the body is relying upon its fat stores for energy. Ketosis induces even more lipolysis to keep the cycle of fat breakdown churning.

This process has several beneficial effects in obesity. Ketosis suppresses appetite, so the individual feels less hungry. Robert Atkins also postulated that ketosis produces a "metabolic advantage," because burning fat for energy takes more calories than burning sugar. Thus, a calorie deficit occurs from both reduced calorie consumption and increased calorie expenditure.

The Atkins diet restricts not only carbohydrates, but also restricts the type of carbohydrates as well as the amount of carbohydrates consumed at any one time. These restrictions have a net effect to keep glucose and insulin levels low, and so maintain the state of ketosis. In place of carbohydrates, the Atkins diet encourages essentially unlimited quantities of protein and fat. While fat intake is not restricted, participants are encouraged to consume no more than 20% of their calories from fat. However, some of the Atkins meal plans have been calculated to contain as much as 63 percent fat. Protein intake has been calculated to provide over 50 percent of the daily calories in some Atkins meal plans.

The only permitted carbohydrates are those with a low "glycemic-index." These are foods that promote a much slower rise in blood sugar, and also insulin, when absorbed into the bloodstream than high glycemic-index foods. The glycemic-index was extensively studied and promoted by Dr. David Jenkins, a physician and nutritionist from the University of Toronto in the 1980s. Jenkins theorized that the entry of sugar into the bloodstream in certain types of foods occurred in quick bursts causing high spikes in blood glucose. This induced an overstimulation of insulin secretion by the pancreas. Over time, this caused cells to become resistant to insulin, and led to even more insulin production. This caused a persistent decline in blood glucose levels, which would initiate a cycle of hunger; excess sugar leads to excess insulin, which leads to low sugar, which leads to hunger, which leads to consumption of more sugar. The resulting insulin resistance and weight increase also promote the development of metabolic syndrome and diabetes.

Foods with a high glycemic-index cause the quick bursts and spikes in blood glucose. Such foods are very prominent in a typical western diet. They often contain processed sugars and heavily refined starches, or naturally have the property of containing high levels of sugar that is quickly absorbed in the gastrointestinal (GI) tract when consumed. The few carbohydrates that are permitted in the Atkins diet are whole grains, cereals, beans and most fruits and vegetables, all of which have a low glycemic-index. Thus, they do not promote sugar and insulin spikes, and reduce the sensation of hunger. A list of these foods is shown in **table 10.2**.

Table 10.2
Glycemic Index of Selected Heart-Healthy Carbohydrates

Glycemic Index	Fruits	Vegetables	Grains	Legumes	Dairy
Low (< 30 %)	Cherries	All except those below		Soy beans Peanuts	Low fat yogurt
Medium (30-50%)	Apples Grapes Peaches Pears Grapefruit Berries Figs Olives	Radishes	Barley Oatmeal Whole rye	Lentils Kidney beans Split peas Lima beans Chickpeas	Milk Fruit yogurt
High (50-80%)	Oranges Plums Kiwi fruit Prunes	Sweet corn Sweet potato Carrots* Beets	All pastas Wheat	Navy beans Pinto beans	Ice cream (low fat)
Very High (>80%)	Apricots Bananas Mangos Papayas Raisins Pineapple Watermelon* Dates	Pumpkin White potato Rutabaga Parsnips	Rice Couscous	Fava beans	Ice cream

All glycemic index values referred to the item in the fresh state, unpackaged and uncooked.
*indicates food for which glycemic load is significantly lower than glycemic index at standard serving amounts.

The Atkins diet proceeds through four phases; each phase becomes progressively less restrictive in carbohydrate intake. The first phase or induction lasts two weeks. During this phase, carbohydrate intake is limited to less than 20 grams per day. This is the phase during which participants typically experience the greatest weight loss, up to five to ten pounds per week. The first appearance of ketosis in this phase induces dehydration, and thus abundant fluid intake is encouraged. No alcohol is permitted during the induction phase. The second phase, called Ongoing Weight Loss

(OWL) permits an additional five grams of daily carbohydrate each week, and lasts until the participant is within ten pounds of their target weight. An additional ten grams is added daily during each week of the third phase, called Pre-maintenance. The final phase is called Lifetime Maintenance, and is intended to be continued indefinitely.

> **Illumination:** In the years 2003–2004, at the height of its popularity, an estimated one in 11 North American adults was on the Atkins diet. Annual sales of carbohydrate foods like pasta and rice declined by 8.2% and 4.6% respectively during these years.

The cardiovascular benefits of the Atkins diet remain a subject of much debate. Some studies conclude that the Atkins diet helps prevent cardiovascular disease, provides metabolic benefits, lowers LDL-C and increases the amount of HDL-C. Other studies have found many patients have significant rises in blood lipids and inflammatory markers on the Atkins diet. A Swedish prospective study with a follow-up of approximately ten years came to the conclusion that elderly Swedish men on a carbohydrate-restricted diet similar to Atkins had a 20 percent increased risk of death from all causes and a 40 percent increased risk of CHD-related death.

Although glucose levels drop in the Atkins diet, the diet does not appear to improve long-term sugar control in diabetics, or reduce the likelihood of developing diabetes. Blood pressure generally drops in individuals in the Atkins diet. However, this may be due to the dehydration that accompanies the induction phase. Some studies suggest that the diet can contribute to osteoporosis and kidney stones as more calcium is excreted through the kidneys. Concerns have been raised regarding consumption of high levels of protein in individuals with medical conditions such as kidney disease or gout.

Nearly all participants lose weight on the Atkins diet. The majority of the weight loss occurs in the first two weeks during induction. The initial weight loss is nearly all due to loss of body fluids induced by ketosis. Multiple clinical studies have demonstrated an average of ten pounds of weight loss within the first month. However, maintenance of weight loss over the subsequent six to twelve months is highly variable, ranging anywhere from none and up to ten pounds.

Comparisons of weight reductions observed in the Atkins versus other diets have also been studied in clinical trials. In nearly all instances, while initial weight loss is greater in the Atkins diet, by one year Atkins participants fare no better than participants in other diet plans.

South Beach Diet. When he introduced the South Beach Diet in the early 2000s, Arthur Agatson was a practicing cardiologist who had already achieved notoriety for his work on developing the CAT scan coronary calcium scoring system (CCS) discussed in earlier chapters. Agatston accepted the prevailing wisdom among cardiologists that a low-fat diet would reduce cholesterol and prevent heart disease but found that in practice, patients had a difficult time sticking to the diet. He also believed in the metabolic principles of the Atkins diet but thought the saturated fat content was too high and the carbohydrate and fiber content too low to provide long-term benefits in the prevention and management of CHD. As a compromise to both diet plans, the South Beach Diet was born.

Agatson postulated that the low-fat diets promoted by the AHA did not work because total caloric intake did not change. Patients following low-fat diets simply compensated for the lower fat intake by consuming additional sugar and simple carbohydrates. This led to cycles of hunger, resulting in an ongoing excess consumption of calories and weight gain as described by David Jenkins in his promotion of the glycemic-index. Thus, Agatson observed that paradoxically a low fat diet often led to an increase in CHD risk caused by overeating, increase in insulin resistance and weight gain.

To break the cycle, in the South Beach Diet, Agatson proposed consumption of both carbohydrates and fats. However, "bad" carbohydrates were replaced with "good" carbohydrates, and likewise, "bad" fats were replaced with "good" fats. Like Atkins, the "good" carbohydrates are those with a low glycemic-index. These take the place of "bad" carbohydrates like baked goods, processed and refined grains and many root vegetables. For fats, the "bad" fats, like trans-fats and saturated fats are either eliminated or restricted to a much greater degree than in the Atkins diet. Unsaturated fats and foods containing omega-3 fatty acids are encouraged as "good" fats.

Like Atkins, lean protein is an important component of Atkins. Thus, lean meats, nuts, oils with omega-9 monounsaturated fats and oily fish with omega-3 polyunsaturated fats are also encouraged.

Agatston divides the South Beach Diet into three phases, and like the Atkins diet, each phase becomes progressively more liberal in permitted carbohydrate intake. Phase one lasts for the first two weeks of the diet. It eliminates all sugars, processed carbohydrates, fruits, alcohol and some higher glycemic vegetables as well. The only allowed foods are ample portions of lean protein, good fats and the lowest glycemic-index carbohydrates. Its purpose is to eliminate the hunger cycle and is expected to result in significant weight loss. Phase two continues as long as the dieter wishes to lose weight. It reintroduces most fruits and vegetables and some whole grains and low amounts of alcohol as well. Most starches and other high glycemic-index carbohydrates are still prohibited. Phase three is the maintenance phase and lasts for life. There is no specific list of permitted and prohibited foods. Instead, the dieter is expected to understand the basic principles of the diet and live by the principles.

Like Atkins, the majority of individuals following a South Beach Diet will lose weight within the first two weeks. Much of the initial weight loss is due to ketosis-induced dehydration. The average early weight loss is eight to thirteen pounds, and after three months the typical individual continuing to follow the diet will be ten to fifteen pounds below their starting weight. There are few studies evaluating maintenance of weight loss at longer intervals.

Scientific evaluations of the South Beach Diet have been limited but generally favorable. Two high quality clinical trials in 2004 and 2005 found participants following the South Beach Diet showed favorable but only modest improvements in blood lipids, blood pressure and blood sugar. In these trials, the LDL-C levels dropped by only four mg/dL, triglycerides by 41 mg/dL and blood pressure by nine mmHg. Blood sugar was not changed in these trials, but data from other studies show that the Hemoglobin A1C levels in patients following a low glycemic-index diet drop by about ten percent. Favorable results in these parameters usually are evident within three months and have been shown to be maintained as long as participants stick to the diet. However, no long-term scientific study has measured the health outcomes or cardiovascular benefits of patients following the diet.

The Mediterranean Diet

One of the oldest and most intensely studied diet plans is what is commonly known as the Mediterranean diet. The diet is so termed because it draws its principles from a style of eating followed in Greece, Italy, France and Spain. It allows a more generous amount of fat than most of the other diets previously discussed, up to 35–40 percent of daily calories. However, almost all of these fat calories are from unsaturated oils. The diet is balanced across healthy groupings of carbohydrates, proteins and fats. It is high in fiber, lean protein, nuts, fruits, vegetables, legumes and healthy fats. It discourages meats, cheeses and most other dairy products as well as sweets.

Several foods are emphasized in the Mediterranean diet. These include olives, which are rich in the monounsaturated, omega-9 fat oleic acid. This is a potent antioxidant and reduces LDL-C and raises HDL-C. Fresh, colorful vegetables are encouraged as most have a low glycemic-index and are both anti-inflammatory and antioxidant. Fresh fruits with a low glycemic-index are also advised. They are also excellent sources of natural Vitamin C and other antioxidants, which keep the arterial wall and endothelial cells healthy. They also provide high levels of potassium, magnesium and calcium, the same chemicals that are encouraged in the DASH diet for lowering blood pressure.

Lentils and other legumes are advocated as sources of lean protein. On a per-serving basis, lentils provide as much protein as meats do, with virtually no saturated fat or cholesterol. However, most proteins derived from vegetables, legumes and/or grains, such as lentils, are "incomplete." That is to say, unlike animal and dairy proteins, which provide a full complement of all essential amino acids, all vegetable/grain/legume proteins, with the exception of soy and quinoa, contain only some of the nine essential amino acids. Essential amino acids are those that cannot be made by the body and need to be consumed in foods.

For example, beans are low in the essential amino acid lysine, while rice is rich in lysine. Thus, beans and rice are complementary proteins; when they are eaten together one gets a full complement of proteins. If one does not ingest a full complement of amino acids during the course of a day, the amino acids that have been ingested go to waste; they cannot be used by the body for typical protein functions. In addition, please note, it is always better to eat whole grains, such as brown rice, as opposed to white rice.

With an appropriate variety of protein-rich vegetables, legumes and grains throughout the day, the body's protein needs can easily be met without the need for fatty meats or dairy products.

Oily fish servings also provide protein and essential omega-3 polyunsaturated fats that raise HDL-C, provide an antiplatelet effect and may reduce the risk of heart-rhythm disturbances. Four to five servings per week are recommended. The consumption of plant omega-3 alpha-linoleic acid from flaxseeds and walnuts is also encouraged.

Whole grains and oatmeal are basic staples in the Mediterranean diet. They have a low glycemic-index and contain the soluble fiber beta-glucan, which has been shown to lower LDL-C as well as provide an antioxidant effect, lower blood sugar and help to control weight. Alcohol in moderation is recommended because of data supporting its role in a reduced risk of CHD events.

The Mediterranean diet has been a subject of relatively intense scientific inquiry. In 1994, the French Lyon Heart Study showed that patients adhering to a Mediterranean diet had a 50–70 percent lower risk of a second heart attack compared to patients following an AHA-style diet. Most recently, these findings were confirmed and extended to patients without known heart disease in 2003 by the GISSI-P Trial conducted on over 11,000 subjects in Italy. The group that followed a Mediterranean-type diet had a 51% reduction in CHD mortality. In the Nurses' Health Study of 84,000 women without heart disease between the ages of 34 and 59 years, subjects following a Mediterranean diet were able to reduce their risk of CHD events and dying by over 30 percent. The most favorable results were observed in the group of women that consumed fish five or more times a week.

In fact, proponents of the Mediterranean diet point to the thousands of patients in numerous clinical trials in support of it, relative to the paucity of clinical data in support of either the vegetarian or low-carbohydrate diet plans. The debate over low fat compared to other diets was intensified in 2006 by the findings of the Women's' Health Initiative (WHI) which reported on the outcomes in an 8-year follow-up of 49,000 American women following a reduced fat diet. The study found no reduction in CHD events, weight loss or the occurrence of common types of cancer.

In addition to the CHD benefits described above, the Mediterranean diet has been shown to produce modest improvements in weight, blood pressure, blood sugar and lipids, at levels comparable to the other diet plans discussed above.

The Mediterranean diet has some disadvantages. The recommended basic foods, such as fish and olive oil, can be expensive. Some of the fresh ingredients may be difficult to find at certain times of the year. Meal preparation may be more complex, compared to meal-replacement or exchange diets. The diet is harder to follow when eating out in restaurants in the United States.

Also, the diet is more a style of eating rather than a formal plan and, as such, may be more difficult to follow. The diet provides no rigid recommendations on calories or nutritional percentages of caloric intake. Weight loss occurs only through achieving a calorie deficit, and not through any metabolic advantage of specific types of foods. However, when combined with an exercise program, participants following a Mediterranean diet lose as much weight as those following other diets in both the short-term as well as in long-term maintenance.

The Best Diet?

Which diet should you follow? The answer depends on several things. What are you trying to achieve? Weight loss, healthier metabolism, improved cholesterol or a reduced CHD risk? Just for the treatment of lipid disorders, a diet that reduces LDL-C may be very different from one that reduces triglycerides. Another consideration: Which style suits you? Can you do without meat, bread, alcohol? Other important questions include: Do you have diabetes, kidney disease, gluten sensitivity, hypertension or other medical conditions? Do you take medications that are affected by diet, like warfarin or certain blood pressure medications? How much can you afford in terms of money, time and effort devoted to the diet?

The answers to these questions, in concert with advice from your health care provider, will dictate which diet you should follow. In my opinion, the easiest diets to follow from the standpoint of expense and ease of access to foods are the nationally endorsed TLC, AHA and DASH diets. The most difficult diets to follow, with respect to a significant change in the types of food from those to which most people in the United States are accustomed, are the Portfolio, Ornish, and Pritikin plans. However, there is substantial data to support these plans' effectiveness in not only preventing and treating CHD, but also in reversal of atherosclerosis. In patients who are unwilling or unable to take medications to lower LDL-C, these diets offer the best evidence of improvement in blood lipids. Furthermore, the Ornish and Pritikin plans also offer complete lifestyle modification plans beyond diet intervention.

The Atkins plan may the most effective means to rapid weight loss among all the diets, but it is also the most controversial with respect to long-standing benefits in metabolism, blood lipids and CHD risk reduction. The South Beach and Mediterranean diets offer good compromises in terms of palatability, familiarity and effectiveness. However, they may be the most expensive and difficult to follow with respect to cost and effort in implementation and maintenance. Also, both are plans more devoted to style and types of foods, rather than specifying caloric goals.

Thus, there may well be no single best diet. As the data above indicates, studies in motivated patients supervised by passionate researchers have found all of the diets discussed above to be of value. Among the medical community of nutrition and weight management, it is commonly said that "diets don't fail, people do." Anybody who has started a diet has found that the initial enthusiasm and motivation wane over a period of time, and maintaining the conviction to follow a diet plan is indeed very difficult. This common knowledge is, in fact, supported by sound scientific observations. A 2005 study comparing four different diet plans in 160 participants found that all four diets yielded comparable results in terms of weight loss, blood pressure, blood sugar, LDL-C, HDL-C, CRP and other CHD risk markers. What was remarkable was that after one year, nearly 50 percent of the participants in each diet plan had dropped out of the study. Those that continued to follow the diet, irrespective of which diet, showed the best results. Thus, success lies more in adherence to the diet, rather than the diet itself.

If drop-out rates in a clinical trial are as high as 50 percent, what are they in the real world of patient care? Certainly much higher. A variety of measures have been found to increase the rates of compliance and adherence to diets. The concept of "buying in" to the program appears to be one of the most important factors in adherence to an eating plan. This means that understanding the principles, believing they will work for you, accepting the compromises and sacrifices required of the diet, and ultimately establishing the diet as a way of life that will improve the quality and longevity of one's life are most important.

Heart-Healthy Foods

In my practice, I encourage patients to use diets to achieve specific short-term goals. This may be to jump-start a weight loss program, initiate aggressive or focused lipid reduction, and improve blood pressure or blood sugar. However, for the long-term maintenance of good cardiovascular health, rather than a specific diet, I encourage patients to make wise food choices. This means avoidance of the unhealthy foods that we discussed in Chapter five and specifically seek out those selections that are on the list of heart-healthy foods.

In fact, there is substantial evidence that specific types of foods, independent of the diet in which they are used, offer cardiovascular benefits. In many cases, simply emphasizing these foods in your diet, as opposed to the unhealthy types of foods we have previously discussed, will improve your heart health without you necessarily following a specific diet plan. In this section we will discuss these foods and the evidence supporting their heart benefits. Keep in mind that while the foods discussed below have proven heart benefits, it is still necessary to control calories, balance nutritional intake and ideally incorporate these foods into an overall wellness plan that meets your individual needs and will help you realize your specific goals.

Fruits. Multiple daily servings of fruit are recommended in most heart-healthy diet plans. They provide a significant boost in blood-pressure-lowering chemicals like potassium, magnesium and calcium. A higher level of fruit intake also helps with weight control. A recent study found that simply by replacing one starch serving with one daily serving of fruit (100 grams), will result in four pounds of weight loss per year. If this is done at every meal, over the course of a year, the results will be a loss of 12 pounds. That is without the effect of any other interventions for weight loss.

Beyond weight and blood-pressure control, there is overwhelming evidence of the anti-atherosclerotic cardiovascular benefits of fruit. Fruits with the most cardiovascular benefits are those with the lowest glycemic-index (**table 10.2**), the highest fiber content, and the highest levels of antioxidants and anti-inflammatory compounds. Caloric intake with most fruits is usually not an issue, as most single fruit servings will be between 25 and 100 calories.

Dietary soluble fiber found in fruits reduces cholesterol and lipids by binding dietary fats into the intestine and thus preventing their absorption into the bloodstream. Between ten and 30 grams daily of soluble fiber is recommended. A single serving of most fruits has between two to four grams of soluble fiber. Fruits high in fiber include apples, bananas, berries, cherries, dates, nectarines, plums, prunes, raisins, peaches, pears and starfruit.

Many fruits are rich in the anti-inflammatory compounds. These chemicals are also known to enhance the health of the important arterial lining layer of cells called the endothelium. Among the best are blueberries, dark grapes, apples, apricots and black currants. Worth noting is that the generation of many anti-inflammatory compounds is stimulated by light. Therefore anti-inflammatory compounds are found in higher quantities in the outer rinds of fruits and vegetables; therefore whenever possible they should be eaten unpeeled to derive the most benefit.

Most fruits are high in many antioxidant chemicals, which negate the oxidation of the LDL particle in the arterial wall, the necessary process by which LDL-C is transformed into arterial plaque. Fruits with high antioxidant content are figs, red grapes, olives (yes, olives are a fruit), pomegranates, apricots and mandarin oranges. Naturally occurring vitamin C has repeatedly been shown to be protective against atherosclerosis. It is the body's main water-soluble antioxidant. Blood levels of vitamin C that are too low triple the risk of a heart attack. Supplementing vitamin C naturally with foods was shown, in a study from Norway, to reduce the progression of atherosclerosis. One reason obtaining vitamin C from foods is preferred to supplements is that vitamin C in the blood is very quickly metabolized. However, when vitamin C is ingested with foods containing anti-inflammatory compounds, its life as an antioxidant is extended. Fruits high in vitamin C include all types of citrus, cantaloupes, guavas, kiwis, mangoes, peaches, papayas, pineapples and strawberries.

Vegetables. Vegetables offer many of the same anti-atherosclerotic benefits as fruits. They are high in fiber, and those with a low glycemic-index and high antioxidant and anti-inflammatory content are the most beneficial. Many vegetables also contain a high quantity of phytochemicals, such as phytosterols, that help lower cholesterol and also work as free-radical scavengers to reduce inflammation and oxidation.

The most heart healthy vegetables come from all different classes, ensuring that it is possible to find selections that meet any individual's palate and cooking style. Virtually all vegetables and herbs have been found to have heart benefits. Some vegetables have unique anti-atherosclerotic properties making them worthy of special mention. Garlic and onions are rich in organosulfur compounds, immediately noticeable by their pungent smell. These vegetables not only boost the immune system but also marginally lower LDL-C. Cauliflower and broccoli do the same thing and also lower blood sugar. Nutritional studies show that green leafy vegetables will lower the risk of diabetes by approximately nine percent for each daily serving consumed. The risk of metabolic syndrome can be cut in half by significant consumption of greens.

Caloric intake with most vegetables is usually not an issue, as most single servings will be between 20 and 80 calories. Keep in mind that those with the lowest glycemic-index, as noted in **table 10.2** should be given preference. They will not only provide the cardiovascular benefits discussed above, they will be the best to help control blood sugar, triglycerides, metabolism and weight.

Whole Grains. Whole grains have been proven to provide cardiovascular benefits. Just the fiber in whole grains can reduce LDL-C. A 2004 pooled analysis of nutritional studies in over 2.5 million adults indicated that for every ten-gram increase in daily fiber intake, the risk of CHD events drops by ten percent, and the risk of CHD death drops by 25 percent. The average American diet contains just 15 grams of total dietary fiber. The recommended total fiber intake based upon scientific data evaluating its benefits is between 25 and 40 grams per day.

Unfortunately, most commercially available grains in the U.S. are refined and processed. These are fundamentally different from natural whole grains. Natural whole grains use the entire seed or kernel of the grain. The seed of any grain, whether it is wheat, oats, barley, rice, corn, etc., consists of the bran fiber in the outer skin, the starch in the center and the inner germ, which contains the most nutritious components of protein, healthy fats, minerals, antioxidants and vitamins. Processed grains remove most of the bran and the germ, and so use only the center starch. This process removes both the fiber and the nutrients.

Oats are an especially beneficial whole grain because they contain the largest quantity of the soluble fiber beta-glucan, which can substantially lower LDL-C. Oats are also very high in antioxidants. Regular consumption of oats has also been proven to lower blood pressure, lower risk of metabolic syndrome, improve diabetes control and reduce weight. Eating oatmeal is one of the best ways to routinely and easily derive the benefits of oats. Oats are also one of the lowest-calorie dense grains. A typical one-third cup serving of oats yields about 100 calories, as opposed to a one-third cup serving of barley, wheat or rice, which will provide about 200 calories.

Lean Protein. Lean protein is a component of all the major dietary programs noted above except the purely vegetarian-based carbohydrate diets. Dietary protein has numerous health benefits in and of itself. The body consumes more calories in digesting protein than it does fats and carbohydrates. To digest 100 calories of protein, your body must burn 25 calories, compared to only ten to fifteen calories to digest 100 calories of fats or carbohydrates. Protein when combined with resistance exercise also increases lean muscle mass and reduces body fat percentage. This makes the body a more efficient utilizer of calories, making it easier to control weight when you are leaner.

> **Illumination:** All else being equal, the preferred carbohydrate ingested should be one with the lowest glycemic-index. Typically, these foods also have the highest fiber content and provide the best metabolic benefit. Glycemic-index is not only a function of the sugar content of the fruit, vegetable or grain, but can also be affected by the fiber and fat content of food, since both can affect how quickly the sugar in the food is absorbed from the stomach.
>
> Many diets support the use of low glycemic load rather than low glycemic-index foods. The glycemic load incorporates the quantity of carbohydrate in the food, along with the quality of the carbohydrate as it relates to how quickly it can be digested and absorbed as sugar into the bloodstream. Some foods with a high glycemic-index actually have a low glycemic load. In this case the food may have its sugar digested and absorbed quickly, but it actually contains a relatively small amount of carbohydrate. This is true for carrots and watermelon, both having medium to high glycemic-index levels but low glycemic loads. Foods with a low glycemic-index always have a low glycemic load. The value of glycemic load as it relates to weight loss, development of diabetes or CHD has not been studied as extensively as glycemic-index. No clinical studies have yet to show that a diet plan based purely upon either low glycemic-index or low glycemic load results in a reduced risk of CHD.

Excellent sources of lean protein are egg whites, fat-free or low-fat dairy products, turkey, fish and other lean meats, and nuts. Eggs with the yolk contain 150–220 milligrams of cholesterol. However, egg whites contain no cholesterol, and are almost exclusively protein. Eggs from chickens fed a vegetarian diet rather than animal fats and animal by-products are also lower in cholesterol, with a content of 140–180 milligrams.

Fat-free or low-fat milk, yogurt, cheese and cottage cheese provide protein with virtually no fat. They are also excellent sources of calcium, potassium, vitamin A and D and are not only heart-healthy but prevent bone loss. The white meat of a turkey is one of the leanest meats you can consume; a four-ounce portion contains only 0.4 gram of saturated fat. Even carefully selected red meat, like a trimmed veal steak can be a good choice; a four-ounce portion contains only 0.75 gram of saturated fat.

Many nuts like almonds are not only good sources of lean protein; they also have monounsaturated fats, fiber and vitamin E. A recent meta-analysis of 25 pooled trials studying the lipid-lowering effects of nuts found a modest daily intake of nuts caused total cholesterol and LDL-C levels to drop by five percent and seven percent respectively, and triglyceride levels to drop by ten percent. The Nurses' Health Study and others have found that eating nuts at least five times per week reduces the risk of death by 35–60 percent. Peanuts and walnuts are also on the list of healthy nuts, as discussed below.

Legumes. Legumes are seed-based vegetables like beans, peas, chickpeas, lentils, soybeans (tofu and edamame) and peanuts. They are an important component of all vegetarian diets, as well as the Mediterranean diet, as they are an excellent alternative to meats as a source of protein. If you use a variety of legumes and vegetables, you can ensure that you will be getting complementary proteins that will provide a balance of all essential amino acids.

There is substantial evidence of the cardiovascular benefits of legumes. This comes not only from studies attesting to the benefits of the Mediterranean diet in general, but a study of over 9,000 healthy individuals followed for 19 years, published in 2001, found that those who consumed legumes more than four times per week had a 22 percent lower risk of cardiac events than those who consumed legumes less than once a week.

Legumes are slightly higher in calories than fruits and other vegetables, typically ranging between 100 and 150 calories per 100-gram serving. However, they offer a high content of protein with virtually no associated fat. For comparable serving sizes, legumes can provide the same amount of protein as meats, and do so with no saturated fat or cholesterol, with a higher quantity of healthy fiber, and with fewer calories.

Like many fruits and vegetables, legumes have a high amount of soluble fiber and most have a low glycemic-index. Thus, they are effective in preventing insulin resistance, metabolic syndrome and treating diabetes. They are also high in antioxidant, anti-inflammatory and endothelially beneficial chemicals. Legumes also provide an excellent source of folate, an important chemical that reduces the amount of the atherosclerosis-promoting amino acid homocysteine. Peanuts are best consumed out of the shell or in natural types of peanut butter. Otherwise the added fat and salt content may negate some of the nutritional benefits.

Monounsaturated Fats. A high intake of monounsaturated fats is recommended by nearly all heart-healthy diet plans other than the traditional vegetable-based Pritikin and Ornish plans. The Nurses' Health Study of 84,000 women followed for 14 years showed that for every five percent increase in total calorie intake from monounsaturated fat, there was a 19 percent drop in CHD risk. Oleic acid from the omega-9 family of fatty acids is the primary fat component of monounsaturated fats. Oleic acid lowers cholesterol, LDL-C and blood sugar. It also is an antioxidant and an anti-inflammatory and raises HDL-C. Excellent sources are olive oil, canola oil and safflower oil, all of which have 60 percent or more of their fatty-acid content from oleic acid.

Olive oil in particular is especially beneficial as it has the benefits of being a fruit as well as having a high content of oleic acid. It has also been noted that olive oil inhibits platelet stickiness, thus reducing the risk of arterial clots. Nutritional studies from Greece and Spain have shown that individuals who consume two to three tablespoons of olive oil per day can reduce their risk of CHD by 50 percent and their risk of MI by 82 percent. In fact, the health benefits of olive oil are so solid that the FDA in 2004 issued a qualified health claim for olive oil that states: "*Limited and not conclusive scientific evidence suggests that eating about 2 tablespoons (23 grams) of olive oil daily may reduce the risk of coronary heart disease due to the monounsaturated fat in olive oil. To achieve this possible benefit, olive oil is to replace a similar amount of saturated fat and not increase the total number of calories you eat in a day.*" Other good sources of oleic acid are avocados and almonds. Both also contain potassium, which lowers blood pressure, as well as the antioxidant vitamins C and E, and fiber and folate.

Alert! Olives and olive oil are more calorie rich than other fruits because of their fat content. A tablespoon of olive oil contains 100 calories and a single olive has five calories. Also, a single avocado has about 300 calories, and a handful of almonds have about 140 calories. So keep these numbers in mind when consuming monounsaturated fats, especially if weight reduction is a priority.

Polyunsaturated Fats. Polyunsaturated fats are also generally heart-healthy fats. The Nurses' Health Study, mentioned above, in which the heart benefits of monounsaturated fats were evaluated, also assessed the impact of a diet high in polyunsaturated fats. Researchers found an even greater benefit to polyunsaturated fat intake, with just a 5 percent increase in calories from polyunsaturated fat resulting in a startling 38 percent drop in CHD risk, twice the benefit that was recognized by an increase in an equivalent amount of monounsaturated fat intake.

There are two types of polyunsaturated fats: omega-3 and omega-6. The body cannot make its own polyunsaturated fat, so it must be obtained from the diet. Omega-3 fats are found in high quantities in seafood as the long-chain fatty acids eicosapentaenoic acid (EPA) and docosahexaenoic acid (DHA). In plants, the major omega-3 is alpha-linoleic (ALA) acid. The major omega-6 fatty acid is linoleic acid (LA).

a. Omega-6. While a polyunsaturated fatty acid, the omega-6 linoleic acid (LA) is pro-inflammatory and when consumed in excess is considered unhealthy for the heart. In fact, LA is closely related structurally to the extremely unhealthy trans-fats. LA is ubiquitous in foods in the western diet. It is found in especially high concentrations in sunflower oil, corn oil, soybean oil and cottonseed oil. LA accounts for 90 percent of the fatty acids in the LDL particle. It is susceptible to free-radical attack and oxidation, thus enhancing the risk of LDL-C being turned into plaque. One study showed that patients with a high level of LA have twice the risk of a fatal MI than those with lower levels.

There is controversy as to the optimal ratio of omega-6 to omega-3 fatty acids that should be consumed. Omega-6 has definite health benefits, especially for the neurological system. It is believed that the optimal ratio of omega-6 to omega-3 is 1:1. The average American diet is estimated to have a 17:1 ratio of omega-6 to omega-3. Thus, conventional wisdom is not that omega-6 is unhealthy but rather that our current dietary omega-6 consumption is proportionally too high, and that omega-3 should be boosted in preference to omega-6.

b. Omega-3 from Fish Oil. The evidence for the cardio-protective effect of omega-3 fatty acids is overwhelming. As early as 1944, scientists observed that Eskimos in Greenland had a very low incidence of heart disease. They consumed nearly 15 grams of fish oil daily. Not only does the evidence from the Nurses' Health Study support omega-3 intake, so does that from multiple other studies, such as the DART and GISSI-P trials, which show fish-oil intake lowers the risk of CHD. Fish intake has also been shown to reverse CHD in a recent study of over 40,000 individuals. Finally, a number of trials have shown that omega-3 supplementation significantly reduces CHD events as well as provides protection against developing CHD. This is discussed further in Chapter 13.

Omega-3 fish oil has been shown to reduce plaque by incorporating itself directly into plaque and changing its structure. When plaque from patients consuming fish oil is examined, it has a thicker fibrous capsule and less inflammation, both making it less likely to rupture. Fish oil also lowers triglyceride levels, raises HDL-C levels, makes platelets less sticky and stabilizes the electrical system of the heart.

Another important cardio-protective substance obtained from fish is vitamin D, which has been shown to be a highly cardio-protective nutrient by suppressing inflammation and blocking plaque growth. A recent report from the Framingham trial showed that patients with low vitamin D levels had an increased risk of CHD events by two-fold over a seven-year follow-up compared to patients with normal vitamin D levels.

The best sources of omega-3 are cold water, deep-swimming fish with darker meat, such as salmon, mackerel, lake trout, herring, sardines and albacore tuna. They contain high amounts of EPA and DHA fatty acids. The former is believed to be more potent and protective than the latter. It is currently recommended that individuals consume three and one-half ounces of oily fish two to four times per week. Caloric content of fish is very low, between 80 and 200 calories per each three and one-half ounce serving. The fattier fish like salmon have the higher caloric content.

Keep in mind that commonly consumed fish like cod, flounder, sole, snapper, haddock, grouper, catfish, halibut, swordfish and rainbow trout have only 10–50 percent of the omega-3 content of the best sources listed above. Thus, the type of fish consumed clearly matters.

Mercury intake is no longer a significant concern, but can be reduced further if fish intake is confined to eating open-ocean, deep-water fish more than freshwater fish.

c. Omega-3 from Plants. The omega-3 fatty acid alpha-linoleic acid (ALA) is found in a variety of plants. Patients with high blood levels of ALA have a 50 percent reduced risk of a fatal CHD event. Patients in the Lyon heart study, following a diet high in ALA-rich foods, had a 73 percent lower risk of MI and a 70 percent lower risk of death than those not on the diet. Thus, the plant omega-3 ALA appears to also offer heart benefits similar to those of animal omega-3.

ALA is also an antioxidant and an anti-inflammatory and improves endothelial health. It lowers LDL-C and reduces platelet stickiness. Common sources of plant omega-3 are walnuts and flaxseed. Walnuts have a high content of antioxidants and vitamin E. Flax is high in soluble fiber and also contains antioxidants. It is recommended that at least four grams of ALA be consumed daily, or about a single handful of walnuts and one and one-half tablespoons of ground flaxseeds. Keep in mind that walnuts, like most nuts, are calorie dense, with 190 calories per ounce. Ground flaxseeds yield about 50 calories per tablespoon.

Alcohol. Sophisticated oenophiles and down-in-the-gutter alcoholics alike tout the health benefits of alcohol. Indeed there is strong evidence that regular, light to moderate alcohol intake reduces the risk of CHD. Death rates from MI are 30–50 percent lower in low to moderate alcohol drinkers.

However, alcohol in only marginally greater amounts is associated with a sharp increase in the risk of many other types of heart disease, including arrhythmias, cardiomyopathy and stroke. If diabetes is not well controlled or high blood triglycerides are present, alcohol intake should be very limited. In fact, when consumed by itself, alcohol causes a much higher spike in blood sugar than if consumed with a meal. This is one reason that it is recommended that wine be consumed with meals for optimal health benefits. Alcoholism is also associated with increased blood pressure, liver cirrhosis and reduced life expectancy. Keep in mind that some studies show that alcohol increases risk of breast cancer, and no amount of alcohol is safe during pregnancy. Alcohol can also interact with many prescription medications.

So what is the right amount? Analysis of the multiple studies evaluating the beneficial and harmful effects of alcohol indicates that 14 grams of alcohol for women and 28 grams for men on a daily basis is considered moderate. For women this is equal to one five-ounce glass of wine, one shot (1.5 ounces) of most hard liquor drinks or one 12-ounce beer. For men, it is twice these amounts. For unknown reasons, the French are more liberal in their alcohol intake guidelines, having defined moderate alcohol consumption as 50 grams in men and 25 grams in women. The French truly live their well-known wine toast … *a votre santé* (to your health)!

The heart benefits of alcohol arise from several sources. Alcohol itself is a vaso-relaxant, increasing the elasticity of arteries and lowering blood pressure. Alcohol makes the platelets less sticky, reducing the risk of blood clots. Alcohol raises HDL-C to help remove cholesterol from plaque. Responses of HDL-C are highly variable, ranging from no change, to up to a 26 percent rise in as little as two weeks. Alcohol also tends to preferentially increase the more protective, large, buoyant HDL particles. Alcohol also contains antioxidants, which reduce the incorporation of LDL particles into arterial plaque.

While the health benefits have been shown for all types of alcohol, red wine in particular appears to offer unique benefits. This may have to do with its high content of two unique antioxidants, resveratrol and procyanidins, both of which have been associated with longevity and a reduced risk of CHD. Red wine has ten times the antioxidant content of white wine. Red wines with the deepest, darkest colors, like Cabernet Sauvignon, Bordeaux, Tannat and Pinot Noir have the highest levels of antioxidants.

Illumination: If you do not drink, the general consensus has been that you should not start purely to derive the health benefit. However, a recent study of almost 8,000 subjects followed for four years offers new insight into this recommendation. The ARIC study reported that new adopters of wine consumption reduced their risk of CHD events by 38 percent, compared to lifelong teetotalers. Thus, a frank discussion with your doctor about your individual medical condition and relative risks and benefits of alcohol consumption should be considered for all individuals concerned about taking measures to prevent and reverse atherosclerosis.

Remember that alcohol can be a significant source of non-nutritional calories, and can thus sabotage weight-loss programs. There is a large variation in the calorie content of various alcoholic beverages. A typical five-ounce glass of red or white wine contains about 125 calories. Champagne is actually lower in calories, at about 100 calories per glass, while sweet dessert wines are much higher, between 200 and 250 calories per glass. The calorie content of hard liquor (rum, vodka, scotch, whiskey, gin) depends on the alcohol percentage or proof, averaging 85 calories for 70 proof liquor and going up from there. Some mixed drinks, like a piña colada, Tom Collins or Long Island iced tea, contain 300 calories per drink. Beer contains about 150 calories per 12-ounce serving, and drops to about 100 calories or less for light beer.

Chocolate. Several studies have shown that eating modest amounts of natural chocolate can reduce the risk of CHD as well as improve survival rate after an MI. This may be because natural chocolate is high in antioxidants. The source of the chocolate as well as the type are very important as most commercially available forms of chocolate are treated by a process of alkalinization to reduce the bitterness. This process also removes most of the antioxidants. Dark chocolate found in cocoa powders, unsweetened baking chocolate and dark chocolate squares without added sugar are the least likely to be alkalinized. Be aware that the caloric content of chocolate is high.

Shrimp. Shellfish such as shrimp has traditionally been thought of as being fairly high in cholesterol. However, the type of sterol in shrimp is fucosterol, a non-cholesterol sterol. This chemical is not absorbed when eaten but actually competes with dietary cholesterol for cholesterol-absorbing sites in the intestine. This decreases the absorption of dietary cholesterol in the same way as phytosterol does when ingested. Thus, shrimp can actually lower blood cholesterol. Furthermore, shrimp contain heart-healthy omega-3 fats and almost no saturated fat. Without drawn butter, shrimp is an excellent choice.

Green Tea. At least two Japanese studies have shown that drinking at least one cup of green tea per day can significantly lower the risk of CHD and MI. It has also been shown to lower blood pressure and LDL-C. Green tea has a higher content of natural anti-inflammatory compounds than black tea, and may be part of the reason why cardiovascular benefits are more prominent with green tea. Green tea and green tea supplements are discussed further in Chapter 12.

Chapter 11
TLC—(Part Two):
The First Steps to Good Cardiovascular Health—Healthy Living

IN ADDITION TO modifying dietary patterns to those that are more heart healthy, therapeutic lifestyle changes (TLC) also include other interventions to reduce the risk of CHD (coronary heart disease) and CHD risk factors. In fact, TLC changes are an integral component of many formal cardiac wellness programs, including those discussed in the previous chapter. TLC interventions include changes in body weight, exercise programs, smoking cessation, stress management, maintaining healthy interpersonal and sexual relationships and managing sleep disorders. In this chapter we will review the roles and methods, along with the postulated and proven benefits, of these components of TLC.

Weight Control

Over 65 percent of Americans, or about 130 million people, are classified as overweight or obese. In just the last 40 years the incidence of obesity in the U.S. population has increased from 13 percent to 31 percent. Being overweight or obese is an independent risk factor for CHD as well as for hypertension, lipid disorders and diabetes.

A weight reduction of as little as 10 to 20 pounds will improve blood pressure, lipids and diabetes. A recent study in prediabetics found that there was a 16 percent drop in the risk for developing diabetes for every kilogram (just over two pounds) of weight loss. The Framingham study showed that a loss of only 15 pounds reduced an individual's risk of developing hypertension by 28 percent. Thus, as prevalent and unyielding as the progression of our society into obesity seems, there is ample evidence that controlling and reversing obesity is an important step in the management of atherosclerosis and CHD.

Abdominal fat, or belly fat, is the most dangerous type of fat. It is scientifically classified as "central obesity" or "visceral fat" and is recognized by the "apple-shaped" body type, in contrast to the "pear-shaped" body type, in which fat distribution is more on the periphery than in the central abdomen. In fact, some studies have suggested that central obesity is the single-best predictor of CHD risk.

The average American has 30 billion fat cells. Fat cells in the abdomen are much more metabolically active than those in other areas. They function almost as if they were a separate gland, releasing hormones, fatty acids and other harmful pro-inflammatory and pro-thrombotic substances. Release of fatty acids from these cells contributes significantly to insulin resistance, metabolic syndrome and the risk of diabetes. Hormones like cortisol are also released by these cells and contribute to high blood pressure, fluid retention and an increased level of circulating stress hormones.

Dietary Approaches to Weight Management. Achieving weight control requires altering energy balance, typically expressed by the equation "calories consumed = calories expended." Weight loss occurs when calories expended exceed calories consumed. Optimally, this is achieved by affecting both sides of the equation, increasing calories expended through increasing daily physical activity, as well as reducing caloric intake through diet. For weight loss, the National Heart, Lung, and Blood Institute (NHLBI) recommend decreasing caloric intake by 500–1,000 calories per day, which will result in an approximate one to two pound weight loss per week and, on average, an eight percent weight loss over six months. A simplified approach for determining an appropriate caloric level for weight loss in individuals who are overweight is based upon a person's initial body weight. The NHLBI guidelines are presented in **table 11.1**.

Table 11.1
Estimating Daily Calorie Needs for Weight Loss

Starting Body Weight (pounds)	Suggested Calorie Intake Levels (calories/day)
150-199	1200
200-249	1200-1500
250-299	1500-1800
300-349	1800-2000
>350	2000

Use your starting body weight to determine the amount of permitted calories per day. By staying within the suggested calorie intake levels, you can expect to achieve a 1-2 pound weight loss per week.

Recommended by the NHLBI and adapted from 2004 American Diabetes Association, North American Association for the Study of Obesity and the American Society of Clinical Nutrition joint position statement on lifestyle modifications.

All of the diet plans discussed in the previous chapter can help an individual achieve weight loss. Some plans are more focused on weight loss than others and offer specific caloric goals for intake and expenditure. Others leave the calculation and implementation of caloric intake and expenditure goals to the individual. Careful tracking of calories consumed and expended has repeatedly been shown to increase the chances of success on a weight loss program. Using online programs or smartphone apps for calorie calculation and tracking in the initial implementation of a weight-loss program can be very useful. Keep in mind that any reduced-calorie diet plan should provide the appropriate balance of nutrients, even at lower calorie levels.

Weight-Control Medications. Testimonials abound for patients who were morbidly obese and achieved dramatic success by following a specific diet and/or exercise plan. However, despite the successes chronicled on the television show *The Biggest Loser*, in the real world, individuals who are moderately obese, with a BMI greater than 35 kg/m², are unlikely to achieve and maintain significant weight loss through diet and exercise alone. It is also at these levels of obesity that the health risks are at their greatest.

> **Illumination:** A 2012 study of 123 post-menopausal women from the Fred Hutchinson Cancer Research Center in Seattle found that those following a calorie restricted diet, who kept a food journal to track exactly what they ate over the course of one year, lost an average of 19 pounds compared to only 12 pounds for women who did not keep a journal, a 37 percent difference. The study also found that dieters who skipped meals actually lost less weight than women who ate regular meals.

For these reasons, a number of prescription medications, in combination with lifestyle modifications, are approved for short-term use in the treatment of obesity. Such medications are best administered under the supervision of a health care provider specializing in medical bariatrics. Typically, candidates for these medications must have a BMI greater than 30 kg/m², or a BMI greater than 27 kg/m² along with other health risk factors, such as hypertension, diabetes or lipid disorders. In such patients, obesity medications may be of value in "jump-starting" a weight-loss program, which can then be sustained through adopting good eating, exercise and lifestyle habits.

There are several FDA-approved medications specifically for the treatment of obesity. One of the most commonly used is Orlistat, marketed as the prescription drug Xenical. It is also available without a prescription in a lower-dosage formulation known as Alii. Orlistat inhibits the intestinal fat-modifying enzyme lipase and so blocks fat absorption in the GI tract. Treatment typically results in five to ten pounds of weight loss over a two to twelve month period of medically supervised treatment. Most patients regain the lost weight once they stop treatment. Orlistat is approved for long-term use, up to two years.

There are two amphetamine-based appetite suppressants approved in the United States for short-term therapy to promote weight loss: diethylpropion, marketed as Tenuate, and phentermine. In addition to suppressing appetite, both also increase the body's metabolism and caloric expenditure. Neither has long-term data to support effectiveness, but in the short-term both have been reported to induce five to ten pounds of weight loss. The drug Phen-Fen, which was a combination of phentermine and another amphetamine-derivate, fenfluramine, was used in the 1990s. After it was implicated in causing heart valve defects, it was removed from the market.

Lorcaserin, marketed as Belviq was approved by the FDA in June, 2012, as the first new drug to treat obesity in 13 years. It works by stimulating a receptor for the brain chemical serotonin, which promotes satiety and reduces hunger. Clinical trials show it will help achieve 10–15 pounds of weight loss over a one to two year period. Its approval had been initially withheld because of concerns that it might increase the risk of cancer.

Several medications approved for non-weight loss indications are used "off-label" to promote weight loss. There is anecdotal evidence that the oral diabetes drug metformin, marketed as Glucophage, can induce three to five pounds of weight loss in both diabetics and non-diabetics. Controlled trials of this medication have yielded conflicting results. It is thought to work by lowering insulin levels, which are elevated in the patient with metabolic syndrome or diabetes. Elevated insulin levels promote the sensation of hunger and so stimulate appetite. The injectable diabetes drug exenatide, marketed as Byetta, appears to have a similar effect. The anti-epileptic drug topiramate, marketed as Topamax, is also used off-label to promote weight loss. It is also used to treat bipolar disorder and migraine headaches.

Weight loss assisted by medications has been shown to result in improved health outcomes. Patients have better blood sugar, blood pressure and lipid control. However, long-term outcomes with respect to a reduced risk of CHD or mortality rates have not been shown. All weight loss medications can have adverse effects in anywhere between 10 percent and 30 percent of individuals. The most common include nausea, dizziness, diarrhea, confusion and insomnia. Orlistat causes mostly GI side effects. It can cause deficiency of fat-soluble vitamins, so vitamin supplementation is always needed. It has rarely been associated with severe liver damage. Diethylpropion and phentermine can also cause high blood pressure and heart-rhythm disturbances. There are numerous risks in using the off-label medications for a purpose for which they have not had extensive study of safety and efficacy and are not approved.

Surgical Treatment for Obesity. Surgical treatment for obesity, commonly referred to as bariatric surgery, is becoming more commonplace. In the mid-1990s, there were only 15,000 weight-loss operations performed in the United States. In 2005, the number was 180,000, and in 2008, it was up to 220,000. The basic operations work in one of two ways; (1) by mechanically restricting the amount of food patients can eat and/or (2) by disrupting food absorption through the surgical removal of parts of the digestive system. Liposuction, in which abdominal fat is surgically excised, is not bariatric surgery.

Candidates for bariatric surgery undergo stringent screening as well as medical and psychological evaluations. Current criteria for candidates are that they must have a minimum BMI of 40 kg/m² for at least five years, or a minimum BMI of 35 kg/m² with significant medical complications related to obesity. Among others, these can include diabetes, CHD or sleep apnea. Recently the FDA has approved the lap-band procedure in patients with a BMI of 30 kg/m² or greater if they also have at least one medical condition linked to obesity. The typical age restrictions are between 18 and 65 years, although this is not set in stone. All patients must have failed traditional, medically supervised weight loss strategies.

Until recently, bariatric surgery was performed only through the "open" approaches, which involved cutting the stomach in the standard manner through a large incision in the abdomen. However, the most common types of operations now are performed laparoscopically. Using much smaller incisions, micro-instruments and video cameras passed inside the abdomen, surgeons can perform most bariatric operations more safely, with much less trauma and fewer complications.

The two most commonly performed procedures that restrict food intake are the adjustable gastric band (AGB) procedure and the vertical sleeve gastrectomy (VSG). Both are performed laparoscopically. The AGB is commonly known as the lap band. In a lap-band procedure, a saline-filled, adjustable bracelet-like band is surgically implanted around the upper part of the stomach to reduce the size of its opening. The constriction created by the band can be adjusted by altering the amount of saline inside the band. At the time of surgery, a small port that connects to the band is placed beneath the surface of the skin in the abdomen. This permits ongoing adjustments of the band after surgery during outpatient visits. These adjustments are painless, and allow the amount of food to enter the stomach to be customized for each patient. The lap band is reversible and causes no permanent change in anatomy. Because the band restricts food intake, the patient feels full sooner. The average weight loss is about 80 pounds over two to three years.

In the VSG, or gastric sleeve, the stomach is reduced to about 15 percent of its original size by surgically removing the large portion of the stomach that follows the major (lower) curve. The open edges are then re-attached, leaving the stomach shaped more like a tube, or the sleeve of a shirt. The procedure permanently reduces the size of the stomach and is not reversible. It has gained popularity because it can now be done in one surgical procedure, whereas previously it required two separate operations. In addition to restricting food intake, as in the lap band, the VSG also removes a large portion of the lower wall of the stomach. This has two beneficial effects. There is less absorptive surface in the stomach; therefore more food passes undigested and unabsorbed into the intestine. The lower wall of the stomach produces the hunger-stimulating hormone ghrelin. When removed, ghrelin levels are much lower, thus reducing the feeling of hunger. Another benefit of the VSG is there is no need for any adjustments of any material placed during surgery, as is the case with a lap band. Finally, the average weight loss following a gastric-sleeve procedure is more than with a lap band, typically about 100 to 120 pounds over one to two years.

Until recently, the Roux-en-Y gastric bypass, also known as a stomach bypass procedure, was the most common type of bariatric operation performed. It is considered a "combined" procedure since it restricts both food intake and absorption. Food intake into the stomach is reduced through the creation of a small stomach pouch separated from the main part of the stomach with a stapling device. The pouch is then connected directly to the middle part of the small intestine. This causes food to bypass the lower stomach and upper intestine to prevent absorption. This procedure can also be done laparoscopically. The average weight loss is 140 pounds over one to two years.

There are other less commonly performed procedures also. This list includes the "restrictive" vertical banded gastroplasty (stomach stapling) and the "malabsorptive" biliopancreatic diversion bypass with duodenal switch. Both have more disadvantages than advantages and are currently performed only in highly select patients. The jejuno-ilieal, or intestinal bypass, operation that was common in the 1980s is no longer performed.

Bariatric surgery has been proven to improve health and life span in multiple studies. Between 50 percent and 60 percent of patients have significant improvements in blood pressure and blood lipids. Over 90 percent of diabetic patients show marked improvement, including many showing complete resolution of their diabetes. The risks of MI and stroke are reduced by 30–50 percent. Several studies have shown significantly lower risks of developing cancer. Overall death rates are 20–40 percent lower in patients having bariatric surgery compared to morbidly obese individuals who are left untreated.

Bariatric surgery is generally safe. The risk of dying during surgery is about one in 1,000 and less than one in 100 within the first 30 days after surgery. Patients at greatest risk are those with a BMI over 50 kg/m^2, the elderly and those with known CHD. Minor, non-life-threatening complications can occur in about 20 percent of patients. Surgical results are typically better in hospitals performing greater numbers of operations.

Illumination: Bariatric surgery using the laparoscopic approach typically costs $30,000–$40,000 and requires on average a two- to three-day stay in the hospital. Many insurance companies now cover this procedure, but many still consider it cosmetic.

Patients who have undergone bariatric surgery have to completely transform their diet and activity habits. Patients typically eat more frequent, smaller meals. They must chew their food slowly and more thoroughly. Highly refined foods, alcohol and sweets are either prohibited or very restricted. High protein intake is encouraged. Those undergoing the Roux-en-Y surgery also have to take calcium, vitamin B$_{12}$ and a multivitamin supplement for the rest of their lives. After successful bariatric surgery, the patient needs to commit to significant efforts in exercise, good nutrition and lifestyle modifications to continue to see favorable results from the initial weight loss that occurs after surgery.

Exercise

It is well established that a program of regular physical activity is an important component of a healthy lifestyle. Regular exercise has been proven to be protective against several chronic illnesses including CHD, hypertension, diabetes, osteoporosis, colon cancer, anxiety and depression. On the other hand, lack of regular physical activity is strongly associated with increased death rates.

The benefits of exercise in reducing CHD have long been recognized. In 1953, a study of workers on London transport buses found that bus drivers who sat all day had twice the risk of heart attacks compared to bus conductors who were up and walking all day. In the United States, a similar study of postal workers found that those who worked in postal offices had twice the risk of heart attacks as mail carriers who walked their routes.

Illumination: Lack of exercise appears to confer the same levels of risk for CHD as do other CHD risk factors such as abnormal lipids, hypertension and smoking. In fact, sitting at a sedentary desk job for 6 hours carries the same statistical CHD risk as smoking 25 cigarettes per day. Despite the overwhelming evidence of the benefits of regular exercise, millions of Americans remain sedentary.

Exercise incorporated into a weight reduction plan has several beneficial effects on metabolism, blood pressure, blood lipids and other CHD risk factors. A recent study in women with metabolic syndrome showed that a plan combining physical activity with diet reduced metabolic syndrome risk factors more than three times better than a treatment plan that used diet without exercise. Typically, regular exercise raises HDL-C by five–25 percent and reduces triglycerides by 10–25 percent. Exercise transforms the more dangerous small, dense LDL particles into the less dangerous large, buoyant type. It also improves body composition by lessening abdominal fat and improves insulin sensitivity and immune function. A 2002 study evaluating interventions to prevent diabetes found that simply exercising reduced the risk of diabetes by 50–70 percent in susceptible patients over a three-year period compared to treatment with diet or diabetes medications alone. Regular exercise makes platelets less sticky, thus reducing the risk of arterial thrombosis and embolism.

Exercise helps to reduce the tone of the sympathetic nervous system. This part of our nervous system facilitates the release of stress hormones. This is the mechanism by which exercise is commonly referred to as helping to "burn off" stress hormones. By reducing adrenaline, blood pressure and endothelial function both improve. The sensitivity of the heart to adrenaline is also reduced, thereby reducing the risk of arrhythmias. Exercise also works in the opposite way; it enhances the tone of the parasympathetic nervous system. This part of our nervous system helps facilitate relaxation responses. In this way, exercise reduces resting heart rate and is thought to be protective against CHD and arrhythmias.

Aerobic Exercise. The current recommendation for exercise to manage body weight is that one engage in at least 60 minutes of moderate-intensity physical activity every day, over and above usual daily activity. If weight loss is a goal, then at least 60–90 minutes of moderate-intensity physical activity is recommended. Moderate-intensity physical activity requires consumption of 200–400 calories per hour for a typical 154-pound person. Such activities include hiking, light yard work, dancing, bicycling, walking (3.5 mph, or about one mile in 17 minutes), golfing while walking and carrying clubs, stretching and light weight lifting. A vigorous-intensity workout requires consumption of 400–600 calories per hour for a typical individual. Such activities include jogging, swimming, aerobics, fast walking (4.5 mph, or about one mile in 13 minutes), basketball, and vigorous weight lifting or yard work. The health benefits of exercise occur no matter if the activity is done in one session, or is broken up into several sessions, as long as the intensity level is maintained.

In order to improve cardiovascular fitness, aerobic activity that elevates and maintains heart rate in the so-called training range is necessary. The training range is the pulse rate that reflects that you are working near maximal aerobic capacity. At aerobic capacity, your body is making the maximal and most efficient use of oxygen in energy metabolism. Any physical activity that boosts your heart rate to between 60 percent and 85 percent of your age-predicted maximum, and maintains it at this level for a minimum of 20 minutes, will result in improved cardiovascular fitness. The more strenuous and prolonged the exercise, the greater the cardiovascular benefits. Keep in mind that certain medications like beta-blockers will affect an individual's capacity to elevate heart rate, and in such patients a training range heart rate cannot be established.

> **Illuminaton:** Scientific studies of exercise physiology have established that training range varies according to age and can be quickly estimated by the formula, 220 − age. Thus, for a 50-year-old man the maximum age-predicted heart rate is 170 beats per minute. Thus, a training range of 60–85 percent of maximal heart rate would be between 102 and 145 beats per minute.

Resistance Exercise. Most exercise programs tailored to cardiovascular prevention and treatment have focused primarily on aerobic exercise. There is increasing evidence that resistance training also has cardiovascular benefits. Although aerobics and resistance training fulfill some of the same goals, such as toning muscles and strengthening major muscle groups, they achieve these goals in different ways. Furthermore, there are fundamental differences between aerobic training and resistance training, and that for the purposes of achieving better cardiovascular health, these differences may be complementary.

Aerobic exercise is a calorie-burning activity; it raises the heart rate and keeps it elevated for a sustained period of time. It requires increased respiration and oxygen consumption. Strength training, on the other hand, is primarily meant to build and develop lean muscle mass. It puts muscles through more wear and tear than cardiovascular activities. It is classified as anaerobic because the working muscles do not require an increase in oxygen consumption. Pumping weights is not the only way to perform resistance training. Calisthenics, Pilates, yoga, circuit training and Cross-fit are all examples of types of exercise that have significant components of dynamic resistance training.

When resistance training is done at high intensity, blood pressure transiently increases, and this may be hazardous to the cardiovascular system. However, the dynamic forms of resistance training that involve moderate resistance and high repetitions with short rests are associated with reductions in blood pressure. Both aerobic and resistance exercise have beneficial effects that lower resting heart rate by equivalent amounts. Improvements in glucose metabolism with strength training have also been shown. Thus, it appears that both resistance training and aerobic exercise offer a strong protective role in the prevention of diabetes. Aerobic exercise appears to be somewhat superior to resistance training in improving blood lipids, but several studies have shown a favorable impact of resistance training on blood lipids, especially when done at high repetitions and moderate workloads.

There are numerous health benefits to resistance training beyond those confined to the cardiovascular system. Substantial improvement in all of the components of musculoskeletal health as a result of resistance training have been shown in sedentary, disabled, young, physically active and very old, frail individuals. The lower lipid benefit of resistance training may be offset by the increased benefit in preserving bone-mineral density compared to aerobic exercise.

One reason strength training is metabolically beneficial is that it builds muscle mass. Muscle burns calories more efficiently than fat. Changing your body composition by replacing just five pounds of fat with five pounds of muscle makes your body burn an extra 250 calories daily just to maintain that extra muscle. In the strategy of caloric balance, this is the equivalent of being able to consume an extra 250 calories guilt-free. Muscle building occurs only with resistance exercise. In fact, when you diet to lose weight, the first type of tissue that the body loses is protein, since it requires the most calories to maintain. Therefore, weight loss without exchanging muscle for fat is not only often unsuccessful, it actually can increase your percentage of body fat.

Despite the well-established benefits of exercise, it is prudent to discuss any new exercise regimen with your health care provider. Exercise has been shown to trigger heart attacks in vulnerable patients. In fact, a recent meta-analysis that pooled the results of 14 different studies that looked at the risks and benefits of exercise found that the risk of heart attack is increased by 3.5 times during exercise compared to periods of inactivity. Still, the absolute risks of a heart attack are very low during exercise and are outweighed by the substantial benefits.

> **Alert!** If you have cardiovascular risk factors, are over the age of 50 and have never exercised, have any symptoms that suggest you are at risk from exercising, have chronic health problems or take medications, it may be prudent to have a cardiovascular evaluation and even a cardiac stress test before beginning an exercise program.

The benefits of exercise are quite tangible. A regular exercise program has been shown to reduce the frequency of angina and episodes of congestive heart failure (CHF) and improve endothelial function in patients with CHD. In patients recovering from a heart attack or from heart surgery, a supervised exercise program is designed within the confines of a cardiac rehabilitation program. In cardiac rehabilitation programs, exercise reduces the risk of recurrent heart attack by up to 80 percent and reduces the risk of death by 30–90 percent.

What about patients without known CHD? A 2005 clinical study showed that a moderate to vigorous exercise regimen done for 60 minutes per day added on average 3.7 years to life expectancy. Perhaps of even more importance is that this exercise regimen will add on average 3.2 years of disease-free life, thus attesting to a better quality of life for a longer period of time, in addition to prolonged life expectancy. Furthermore, multiple studies confirm that even a midlife increase in physical activity confers improved longevity, upholding the principle that it is truly "never too late to start."

Smoking Cessation

The health hazards of smoking are well established. Equally well known are the health benefits of smoking cessation. Stopping smoking before the age of 30 restores life expectancy to what it would have been had the individual never smoked. Stopping smoking while in one's 60s can still add three years of a healthy life.

Tobacco contains the chemical nicotine. The addiction to tobacco is primarily a chemical addiction to nicotine. There may also be other addictive factors that affect the ability to stop smoking, including a significant psychological addiction. Tobacco cessation can lead to symptoms of nicotine withdrawal, including anxiety, irritability, depression, insomnia and tobacco craving. These symptoms typically last between one and two weeks.

A common occurrence with tobacco cessation is weight gain. The average weight gain due to smoking cessation is about six pounds in men and eight pounds in women. This is believed to occur because smoking suppresses appetite, and because nicotine is a stimulant, causing increased calorie burning. The increased appetite associated with tobacco cessation may persist for several weeks.

While there are a number of methods to assist in tobacco cessation, the vast majority of smokers quit without assistance. They do this either "cold turkey" or gradually reduce their cigarette intake. Patients who are advised by their doctor to stop smoking are 20 percent more likely to do so than those who receive no medical instructions to stop. Counseling for ten minutes or more will result in a 20 percent smoking cessation rate, double that of patients receiving no counseling. Remarkably, 20 percent of smokers over the age of 50 have never been counseled to stop smoking by their health care providers.

Assisted Cessation. Smoking cessation assisted by medicines is more effective than unassisted cessation. The most common medical treatment is through nicotine replacement therapy. This can take the form of nicotine skin patches, which are available without a prescription, nicotine gum, lozenges, sprays and inhalers. The effectiveness of the nicotine replacement therapies in promoting long-term smoking cessation is seven to ten percent.

> **Illumination:** Community and public policy programs enhance the likelihood of tobacco cessation. Smoke-free workplaces and zones increase smoking cessation rates by 12–38 percent. A ten percent increase in tobacco prices promotes an additional three to five percent of individuals to stop smoking.

There are two FDA-approved prescription medications to assist in smoking cessation. One is bupropion, marketed under the name Zyban. This medication is also used as an antidepressant. The other is varenicline tartrate, marketed under the name Chantix. Both decrease the urge to smoke and also reduce withdrawal symptoms. Smoking cessation rates with these medications range between 25–35 percent, or about twice as high as unassisted smoking cessation. Varenicline tartrate may cause psychiatric side effects, including nightmares and suicidal thoughts. Recently, it has also been associated with an increased risk of cardiovascular events, including MI, CHF, sudden death and arrhythmias.

A number of alternative approaches to smoking cessation have also been touted, with varying degrees of success. These include acupuncture, aromatherapy, hypnosis, herbal therapy, biochemical feedback and the electronic cigarette. In general, these have not been shown to have cessation rates that surpass unassisted cessation. However, they are worth trying in patients who have repeatedly failed unassisted cessation and who are not candidates for cessation medications, as aside from cost, they offer little downside.

Stress Management

Both acute and chronic stress have been shown to hasten the development of CHD and increase the risk of MI and stroke, as well as adversely affect recovery of patients who have already had an MI. Most studies evaluating the benefits of stress reduction in heart disease have been in patients with established CHD who are undergoing short-term cardiac rehabilitation following an MI or heart surgery. Highly structured, long-term programs that incorporate behavioral skills training and focus on stress management of emotional factors have been shown to reduce the risk of recurrent heart attacks by up to 30 percent and the risk of death by nearly 35 percent. These programs have several components, including education, development of self-monitoring skills to recognize stress, cognitive restructuring to alter how one mentally copes with stress, spiritual development and development of tangible stress-management skills to handle stressors such as time, urgency and/or hostility. However, these programs require a long-term commitment, typically bi-weekly, one to two hour sessions over the course of a year. Programs that are less structured or intensive have been shown to have lesser or no significant benefits. Many are not covered by standard health insurance plans.

> **Illumination:** Simply laughing more has been shown to be beneficial to your arterial system. In 2005 researchers measured endothelial reactivity in volunteers who were shown a violent movie and compared their results to those watching a funny movie. Arterial blood flow was improved in most subjects when they laughed during the funny movie and was reduced in most subjects when they perceived stress during the violent movie.

In the prevention of heart disease there are only a handful of trials evaluating stress-reduction interventions, most of which suffer from lack of a uniform approach for managing stress, a short-term follow-up time and small numbers of subjects. Both the Ornish and Pritikin wellness programs include stress-management as an integral component. A number of clinical trials in small groups of patients were recently pooled together in an attempt to assess their effects to prevent CHD. The results of this "meta-analysis" suggest that psychological interventions that specifically target altering Type A behaviors and depression can reduce the risk of developing heart events by up to 20 percent. Methods that offer education about risk factors, group discussions and emotional support groups or aim to involve family members in education and support are less effective than behavior-modifying trials. Most insurance plans also do not cover stress management programs for the prevention of CHD. Thus, most individuals are left on their own to address stress-management.

One proven method to reduce psychological stress is by adopting an exercise program. Thus, benefits in physical and psychological well-being may be achieved simultaneously. Other techniques, such as mediation, yoga and massage may be effective. For many people, channeling stress through recreational activities and hobbies may also be an effective alternative. If Type A behaviors are an important component of one's personality, one should seek counseling to learn adaptive techniques and behavior modification. If stress is associated with depression, as is often the case, antidepressant medication may be of value.

Marriage and Sexual Activity

There is ample evidence that poor interpersonal relationships, and in particular bad marriages, are a major cause of stress. A number of large studies attest to the fact that bad marriages directly contribute to CHD. A study of over 9,000 British civil servants followed over 12 years found that those with the worst marriages had a 34 percent greater likelihood of having heart attacks than those with good marriages. Even after considering other CHD risk factors such as hypertension, obesity and smoking, the quality of the marriage relationship still predicted the risk of developing CHD.

A number of other studies have found strong associations between a healthy marriage and CHD. A 2006 study from the University of Utah of 150 married couples used coronary artery CAT scans to look for CHD. Those couples who behaved with hostility toward each other had more severe calcium buildup in their coronary arteries than couples in good relationships. Studies of women in unhappy marriages reveal that those women who stay silent during marital arguments have a higher risk of dying than women who more readily express their feelings.

> **Illumination:** For men, just being married confers almost a two-fold protection against CHD and death compared to men who are single. For women, being married does not appear to offer any survival benefit over being single, at least as far as the risk of CHD goes.

For men, the amount of sexual activity in their marriage also appears to be inversely related to their risk of CHD. The 2010 Massachusetts Male Aging Study followed over 1,000 men in their 50s who had no evidence of CHD when they entered the study. Over a 16-year period of follow-up, the results showed that compared to men who reported sexual activity at least two or three times per week, men who engaged in sexual activity once per month or less were 45 percent more likely to develop CHD. Similar findings were noted by British researchers who followed 900 men over 20 years. Whether these findings represent better overall general health in men having more frequent sex or better marriages and less stress in men having more frequent sex is not known. Interestingly, among the women in these same studies, there was no observed relationship between the frequency of sex and a reduced risk of CHD.

Risks of Sex. Sexual activity in patients with CHD is generally safe but not completely without risk. The magnitude of the risk of a heart attack during or immediately after sexual activity is about three times higher than at other times. Still, the absolute risk is quite small. A 1996 study reported that in healthy individuals without a history of heart disease, the chance of sexual activity causing a heart attack is about two in a million. The risk rises in people with a history of a prior heart attack, to about 20 in a million. This risk can be lowered in patients with CHD who exercise regularly.

Sexual arousal clearly puts stress in the cardiovascular system. It increases heart rate, blood pressure, breathing rate and oxygen consumption. The energy expended in sexual activity has been calculated to be equivalent to moderately-paced walking. Even the most physically demanding sexual activity will not exceed the effort needed to climb two flights of stairs. Therefore, if walking at a moderate pace or climbing stairs does not cause chest pain, shortness of breath, dizziness, palpitations or fainting, the patient is likely safe to engage in sexual activity. If the patient has known CHD, angina or risk factors requiring medications, it is always safest to ask your health care provider for guidance.

Certainly patients who are recovering from a heart attack, heart surgery, angioplasty or the insertion of stents have unique sexual issues. While sexual dysfunction is common after such events, it is most often due to psychological causes such as loss of libido, anxiety, and depression, rather than physical causes due to underlying circulation problems. It is also prudent to exercise precaution in resuming sexual activity after these events. Usually men and women can resume sex within a few weeks and sometimes in only a few days. In some cases an exercise stress test can not only provide medical guidance, it can also be reassuring psychologically to the patient and his or her partner about the safety of sexual activity.

A recent study from the University of Chicago demonstrated that after suffering a heart attack, only about half of men and a third of women received discharge instructions regarding sexual activity. In the year following a heart attack, fewer than 40 percent of men and 20 percent of women talked with their doctors about sex. However, those who did were 30–40 percent more likely to resume sexual activity after the heart attack.

Sexual Dysfunction. Sexual dysfunction can be a sign of circulatory disorders. In particular, the same PVD (peripheral vascular disease) that occurs when arterial blockages reduce blood supply to the legs can also affect blood supply to the pelvic organs. For men, this can be a cause of failure to achieve and maintain an erection, commonly known as erectile dysfunction, or ED. For women, the symptoms may be more subtle, such as reduced lubrication, painful intercourse or failure to achieve orgasm.

Over a five-year period, men with ED have a 50 percent chance of having an MI or being hospitalized for CHD. On the other side of the coin, 50 percent of all men with CHD will develop ED. Thus, all men with ED and women with sexual dysfunction should be assessed for CHD risk factors and evidence that they may have CHD. ED in men is more likely to be psychogenic if spontaneous and morning erections continue to occur, or if the ED coincides with the occurrence of a significant stress-provoking event.

Sexual dysfunction in men and women can be caused by medications. These include tranquilizers and antidepressants. Many medications used to treat CHD and CHD risk factors like blood pressure medications, anti-arrhythmic medications and nitrates can cause sexual dysfunction.

Drugs to treat sexual dysfunction are being used increasingly in men and women. In general, such medications are quite safe. For women who are post-menopausal, the use of topically or vaginally inserted estrogen poses no increased risk. Female hormones (estrogen therapy) usually do not improve sex drive for women. However, they may promote vaginal lubrication and make intercourse less painful for women who are post-menopausal or who have low estrogen levels. Hormone replacement therapy carries additional risks for women that need to be considered; they are discussed further in Chapter 14.

ED medications like Viagra, Levitra and Cialis are used by millions of men and generate almost five billion dollars in revenue for drug companies worldwide. These medications work by increasing blood flow to the penis. Response rates to ED range from between 50 percent and 80 percent. Headaches, flushing and nasal congestion are common side effects. Cardiac side effects are, however, rare. Nevertheless, such drugs should not be used if the patient is on nitrates for angina or certain blood pressure medications known as alpha-blockers (Cardura, Hytrin, Catapres) or has frequent episodes of angina. Also, patients with heart failure, low blood pressure and those on multiple medications may be at increased risk of side effects.

Other treatments for sexual dysfunction also exist. These include topical methods, mechanical methods, herbs, supplements, antidepressants and penile implants. Patients should always consult with their health care provider before they start any of these treatments. If testosterone levels are low, testosterone replacement may help restore sex drive and libido and correct ED. Testosterone replacement is discussed further in Chapter 12.

Sleep Patterns

Not only are sleep disorders prevalent in the general population, they are associated with a higher risk of developing both CHD risk factors and CHD itself. It is well established that chronic sleep loss increases the risk of hypertension, diabetes and obesity. There are multiple postulated causes related to changes in hormones and chemicals in the body and brain as to why this occurs. There also appears to be an association between sleep deprivation and obesity. Sleep deprivation alters the levels of the hunger hormone leptin. A recent University of Chicago study found that sleep-deprived individuals developed low leptin levels, and those with the greatest drops in leptin levels felt the hungriest. When awake, these individuals ate more than those with normal leptin levels. They particularly craved carbohydrate-rich foods, like ice cream, pasta and bread.

Multiple studies have confirmed that the optimal amount of sleep for cardiovascular health appears to be between seven and nine hours per night. A study from the University of Warwick followed 470,000 participants worldwide over a period of between seven and 25 years. Sleeping less than six hours per night increased the risk of developing or dying from CHD by 48 percent. There was also an increased risk of developing or dying from a stroke by 15 percent. People who reported sleeping more than nine hours per night also had poorer outcomes, but in these cases the excessive sleeping appeared to be a sign of, as opposed to a cause of, cardiovascular problems.

A 2010 study from West Virginia University of 30,000 adults confirmed and extended these findings. Compared to individuals sleeping seven hours per day, those who slept less than seven hours per day, including naps, were at an increased risk for CHD, and if sleep was for five or less hours per day, the risk of CHD was doubled in patients under 60 years old and tripled in patients older than 60. Individuals sleeping over nine hours per day were at one and a half times greater risk of CHD.

It is believed that about 50 percent of simple sleep problems are related to life stress. Work-related issues, followed by family and children concerns are common causes of sleep problems. Recognizing and addressing causes of stress and minor behavior modifications can often have dramatic effects in improving sleep patterns. Some of the recommended strategies are shown in **Table 11.2**. More severe sleep disorders associated with other pathologic responses or dangerous levels of stress may require professional interventions.

Sleep Apnea. One very common sleep disorder linked to heart disease is sleep apnea. In this condition, patients suffer from repeated obstruction of the throat and upper air passages. Their sleep is fragmented and of poor quality, as they must wake up to breathe. Most patients do not recall waking up, but they frequently report nightmares, ongoing fatigue even after a night's sleep, daytime somnolence and snoring.

Table 11.2
Simple Strategies for Modifying Stress and
Helping to Restore Normal Sleep Patterns

- Scheduling time to work through stress and distractions several hours before bedtime, so they do not linger as you prepare to go to sleep.
- Meditation before bedtime.
- Engaging in daily exercise to burn off stress hormones. However, this should not be done within the four hours before bedtime.
- Avoiding caffeine and other stimulants before bedtime.
- Avoiding alcohol within four hours of bedtime. While alcohol is a soporific that may make it easier to fall asleep, it actually interrupts and fragments sleep.
- Taking a warm bath and listening to relaxing music before bedtime.
- Avoiding watching TV before bedtime.
- Keeping regular sleep hours to maintain your biological clock on the same schedule. Go to sleep and wake up at the same time, even on weekends.

Sleep apnea is believed to afflict up to 20 million Americans. Many patients are unaware they have sleep apnea, and only a small percentage receive adequate treatment. Sleep apnea is strongly linked to obesity, and like the chicken and egg, it is not clear whether obesity contributes to the apnea or if the apnea contributes to the obesity. If suspected, the diagnosis can easily be confirmed through an overnight test that can be performed at home or in a medical sleep laboratory called a sleep study.

Sleep apnea increases the risk of hypertension, stroke, heart arrhythmias and MI. This is likely mediated through the effects of increased adrenalin, which is stimulated by a lack of oxygen in the blood during periods of apnea. A recent study of 1,500 individuals followed over four years with moderate to severe apnea found that such patients were at a three to four times higher risk of stroke than patients without sleep apnea. Another study, from Boston University, of 4,500 adults followed for eight years, found that men with obstructive sleep apnea were 58 percent more likely to develop CHF than men without sleep apnea. The risks were greatest in men over the age of 70, who were also at increased risk of MI and CHD. Mysteriously, women with sleep apnea did not show the same elevated risk.

Sleep apnea improves with weight loss, and this remains the primary mode of treatment. Surgeries to widen the air passages or special oral appliances that keep the airway from collapsing have also been effectively used to treat sleep apnea. Sleep apnea is considered one of the medical complications of obesity that qualify a patient with an elevated BMI to be a candidate for bariatric surgery.

Breathing masks that deliver continuous positive airway pressure (CPAP) effectively relieve most apnea episodes by maintaining oxygen flow in the breathing passages under high pressures that prevent collapse of the airways. A recent study using CPAP therapy in 86 patients with moderate to severe sleep apnea found that the therapy reduced blood pressure, cholesterol and the risk of metabolic syndrome and insulin resistance.

Chapter 12
Non-Pharmacologic Therapy for CHD:
The Natural Stuff

NATURAL SUPPLEMENTS AND vitamins are used by 60 percent of all Americans, who collectively spend $20 billion annually on such treatments. In some cases supplements can be an excellent source of bioactive compounds that may be a valuable adjunct to both therapeutic lifestyle changes and traditional medication and surgical therapies for CHD (coronary heart disease). There is a robust body of scientific data in support of a number of bioactive compounds as being valuable in helping to prevent, treat and reverse CHD. Keep in mind that the majority of these bioactive compounds can be obtained from natural foods, and in most cases this is preferable to consumption in tablet form. This is the position of many scientific and national policy bodies like the AHA and the Institute of Medicine.

There are multiple advantages of obtaining vitamins and supplements naturally through foods. Most foods rich in beneficial bioactive compounds are also good sources of fiber. Foods also provide multiple beneficial chemicals packaged together instead of just one specific chemical. Thus, obtaining vitamins and supplements through foods permits a synergistic effect of such chemicals working together to enhance health in the way nature originally intended. In many instances, the absorption of various chemicals is enhanced when they are consumed in foods. This is particularly true of fat-soluble vitamins, which are better absorbed when consumed with fat. Finally, vitamins and supplements can be expensive. They are not covered by pharmaceutical benefit plans, and so all costs are out of your pocket. If you were to take all of the 31 supplements discussed in this chapter at the maximal doses, you would spend ten thousand dollars for a one-year supply!

Dietary supplements provide nutrients, minerals, concentrated metabolites, fatty acids or amino acids that may be missing or not consumed in sufficient quantities in a person's diet. They are under the regulation of the Food and Drug Administration (FDA) as foods and not as drugs. As such, the standards for claims regarding safety and efficacy of a product are not the same as they are for pharmaceuticals. Dietary supplements are permitted to make broad claims supporting structure or function without sound scientific data. For instance, the claim that "glucosamine helps support healthy joints" is permissible, even though there may be no documented benefits of glucosamine preventing or treating arthritis or joint pain in any controlled scientific clinical trial.

Since 2007, the FDA has required manufacturing standards that ensure quality production, packaging and distribution standards to minimize contaminants and impurities, as well as to ensure accurate labeling. However, it is the responsibility of the FDA to verify that the standards are met. It has been reported that between 25 percent and 50 percent of random testing of supplements and vitamins have revealed inaccuracies in their labeling.

Illumination: Unlike the hundreds of pharmaceuticals that have been withdrawn from the U.S. market, only one supplement has ever been required by the FDA to be removed from the market. The weight-loss supplement ephedra was pulled because of its abuse potential and the risk of heart problems associated with its use. This occurred despite significant opposition from the supplement industry and their lobbyists in the U.S. Congress.

A vitamin is an organic compound that cannot be synthesized in sufficient quantities by an organism and so must be obtained from the diet. The term vitamin derives from the words *vital* and *amine*, meaning "nutrient of life." By convention, there are 13 recognized vitamins for humans. There are four fat-soluble vitamins (A, D, E and K) and nine water-soluble vitamins (eight B vitamins and vitamin C). Water-soluble vitamins are not readily stored by the body and need to be consumed daily. Fat-soluble vitamins are more easily stored in body fat and can be replenished intermittently. Like supplements, vitamins are also classified and regulated by the FDA as foods and not drugs.

For all of the reasons noted above, extreme care should be observed in selecting and using supplements for health benefits. It is always best to discuss their use with your health care provider to determine the safety and suitability of any supplement or vitamin in your specific situation. In this chapter we will cover the major over-the-counter (OTC) supplements and vitamins that have been used in CHD prevention, treatment and reversal.

This section is organized so that we discuss those supplements and vitamins that have the most scientific evidence to support their value and safety first, and then move on to those with less evidence of benefit later. For each bioactive compound, the general daily dose range studied for cardiovascular benefit, as well as the current approximate annual cost over the range of specified doses at a discount pharmacy are both noted. In some cases, the compound has a prescription formulation also available, which is so indicated by the designation "Rx available."

"This Stuff Works:" Definitely Effective and Safe

These compounds have significant evidence from either well-designed clinical trials or an analysis of multiple trials, using the meta-analysis methodology, of their likely benefit in preventing, treating or reversing CHD. There may be additional health benefits as well. They are generally safe, affordable and commonly available in OTC formulations. Several also have the support and endorsement of national scientific and public policy bodies. The annual cost of taking the six supplements in this section, at the most common doses recommended for CHD prevention, would be about three hundred dollars.

1a. Omega-3 Fatty Acids: Fish Oil (OTC 1,000–4,000 mg/day, $40–200/year; Rx available). Consumption of omega-3 fatty acids from fatty fish is an important component of many heart-healthy diet plans. There is strong evidence that additional fish oil supplementation is of benefit in both preventing and treating CHD. Of all of the possible supplements available, fish oil is the only one that has received endorsement from all national organizations involved in cardiovascular policy. In 2004, the FDA gave "qualified health status" to omega-3 fatty acids, stating that there was supportive but not conclusive research that they may reduce the risk of CHD.

There are multiple known benefits of consuming fish oil. For blood lipids, fish oil has been shown to reduce triglycerides and Lp(a) and to increase HDL-C. In patients with high triglyceride levels, the maximum dose of four grams per day will reduce VLDL and triglycerides on average by 45 percent. Other benefits in the artery include reducing inflammation, improving endothelial function of the cells lining the arterial wall and promoting plaque stabilization, which reduces the risk of plaque capsule rupture. In one study of 465 women, achieving high blood levels of omega-3 correlated with evidence of less LDL particle oxidation, the necessary step before LDL cholesterol is incorporated into arterial plaque.

Decreasing platelet adhesiveness and stabilization of the heart's electrical system, thus reducing the risk of arrhythmias, are other documented benefits. Regular consumption of omega-3 has also been shown to reduce blood pressure by 4–6 mmHg. It has recently been demonstrated that fish oil also reduces the risks of metabolic syndrome and diabetes.

Fish oil doses and omega-3 content are highly variable among various supplements. The preferred formulation should contain the two major omega-3 fatty acids, eicosapentaenoic acid (EPA) and docosahexaenoic acid (DHA). The recommended total content of these two omega-3 fatty acids per capsule is at least 850 milligrams, irrespective of the total amount of stated fish oil content. These doses are equal to the EPA and DHA content in Lovaza, the oldest and most widely studied prescription formulation of fish oil in the United States.

Numerous clinical studies now attest to the benefits of fish oil supplementation. In patients with known CHD, the GISSI-P Study found that just one capsule per day of fish oil reduced the risk of recurrent heart attacks in Italian patients already having had a heart attack. When combined with statin therapy, fish oil promoted a 20 percent further reduced risk of CHD in Japanese patients with CHD, when compared to statin therapy alone.

For patients without known CHD, a 2007 Japanese study of men with high blood sugar who were administered only EPA fish oil found less plaque and intimal thickening as well as improved blood flow in the carotid arteries compared to those not receiving EPA. Two review articles in 2006 evaluated all published studies of fish oil. Both concluded that scientific evidence supported the premise that regular fish oil consumption was associated with reduced mortality and CHD events.

Illumination: Krill oil is a newly discovered source of omega-3 in marine life. Although limited in scope, evidence supports the fact that krill oil is similar to fish oil in its cardiovascular benefits. It may have fewer GI side effects as it has a lower dose of EPA and DHA. However, krill oil is also more expensive than fish oil, and its lipid lowering effect may be less than standard fish oil.

Side effects related to fish oil are primarily GI in nature. It can cause a fishy odor to the breath, indigestion and diarrhea. These side effects can be prevented or lessened by keeping the fish oil capsules in the freezer and consuming them while still frozen. This causes the capsules to dissolve in the lower intestinal tract, instead of the stomach, and thus reduces some of the side effects.

Mercury contamination in fish oil preparations was at one time a concern. Recent data indicates neither fish oil supplements nor prescription formulations contain significant amounts of mercury. Another potential problem attributed to fish oil preparations was an increased risk of bleeding, by virtue of their blood-thinning properties. A recent report indicated that there was no increased risk of bleeding in patients taking up to seven grams of fish oil per day. Furthermore, a recent study of 610 patients who had CABG heart surgery, and compared subjects who received fish oil alongside other blood thinning medications and those just on blood thinners, found no increased risk of bleeding. In fact, there was a 25 percent reduced risk of bypass graft closure at one year in patients who received fish oil supplements.

1b. Omega-3 Fatty Acids: Flaxseed (OTC 40–50 gm/day, $100–500/year). Flaxseed is an excellent source of plant omega-3 fatty acids. The primary plant omega-3 acid is alpha-linoleic acid (ALA). However, ALA has not been shown to have the same cardiovascular benefits of EPA and DHA (found in omega-3 fish oil). A large clinical trial published in 2002 found no CHD benefit from ALA supplementation. One reason is that ALA has to be converted in the body to EPA and DHA. The average conversion rate of ALA to EPA and DHA is five to ten percent, but it is highly variable from person to person depending on age, sex and metabolism. Women typically have higher conversion efficiency than men.

Consumption of two tablespoons of natural ground flaxseeds is the recommended amount. This provides 40–50 grams of flaxseed. Ground flaxseed has a short shelf life and is prone to oxidation. Therefore, it requires refrigeration to protect it from becoming rancid. Also, while almost 60 percent of the major fat component of natural flaxseed is the healthy omega-3 fatty acid alpha-linoleic acid (ALA), it also has nearly 20 percent of the unhealthy and pro-inflammatory omega-6 linoleic acid. In addition to supplying the health benefits of omega-3, flaxseed also contains fiber, which in selected individuals can also lower LDL by eight to 18 percent. There are few studies evaluating the clinical benefits of natural flaxseed or flaxseed supplements in prevention, treatment or reversal of CHD.

While flaxseed is also available as a supplement, the ALA it contains still has to be converted in the body to EPA and DHA. The supplement also does not provide the fiber found in the natural variety of ground flaxseeds, which may partially contribute to its LDL-C lowering effect. Most supplements are packaged in doses of no greater than 1,000 milligrams, so you would have to take at least 40 tablets to get the recommended amount of omega-3s by supplement. Thus, the natural variety of flaxseed is preferred to the supplement.

Even better than natural flaxseed or supplements are walnuts, which are an excellent source of plant omega-3. Eating just six walnuts will provide the same amount of plant omega-3 as the recommended amount of flaxseed supplement or ground flaxseed. However, walnuts are still not as good as omega-3 from fish, as you would have to consume 36 cups of walnuts to get the equivalent amount of DHA that occurs in three ounces of salmon. Thus, for most people, the preferred source of omega-3 should be fish and fish oil supplements.

2. Phytosterol (OTC 2–3 gm/day, $150/year). Sterols are bioactive substances found in many plants that are chemically similar to cholesterol, hence the suffix "-sterol." By virtue of their chemical structure, once ingested, plant sterols, or phytosterols, interfere with the absorption of dietary cholesterol by blocking the receptors for cholesterol in the intestine. Since these compounds are not actually cholesterol, they are neither absorbed nor used by the body for the manufacture of lipoproteins.

Phytosterols are found naturally in nuts, seeds and vegetable oils. Since the quantities are quite small in these foods, many foods are enriched with sterols. Some of these foods include most margarine spreads, Benechol and some milk products. Numerous studies have shown that eating more plant-sterol enriched foods lowers total cholesterol and LDL-C. In a study of 194 adults with moderately high cholesterol, participants consuming two servings per day of low-fat milk that was plant sterol enriched reduced their LDL-C by nine and one-half percent within three weeks.

The most effective way to obtain plant sterols is as nutritional supplements. Supplements are available as either powders or capsules. Phytosterol supplements are a component of the TLC diet plan and are endorsed by the NCEP. Combined with a low-fat diet, they can reduce total cholesterol and LDL-C by 10–20 percent without the need for prescription medications.

> **Illumination:** Plant sterols also work synergistically with statins. Combining plant sterol with statin therapy may be as effective in LDL-C lowering as increasing the dose of the statin. Taking a low-dose statin plus plant sterol supplement can reduce LDL by an additional 20 percent compared to just statin therapy alone.

3. Green Tea (OTC extract 150–750 mg/day, $70/year; tea 2–3 cups/day, $30/year). The health benefits of drinking green tea have been reputed in the Far East and Indian subcontinent throughout the ages. It is listed in our group of heart healthy foods in Chapter 10. There has been recent enthusiasm for green tea consumption as well as the use of the extract as a health supplement in western society by virtue of clinical studies that seem to confirm the health benefits.

Green tea is derived from the leaves of the *Camellia sinensis* plant, as are the other major teas, black and oolong. Green tea is prepared from unfermented leaves, as opposed to the partially and fully fermented leaves in oolong and black tea, respectively. The absence of fermentation preserves the antioxidant properties of green tea. The caffeine content of green tea is also lower, as fermentation increases the amount of caffeine. Thus, green tea has ten times the antioxidant content and one-third the caffeine content of black tea. The higher antioxidant content also gives green tea a more bitter flavor.

The primary antioxidants in green teas are called catechins, the most active of which is the family known as epigallocatechin-3-gallate, or EGCG. These compounds are scavengers of the free-radical chemicals that can damage DNA and promote lipid oxidation. They work in the same way as the other antioxidants we have discussed that are found in alcohol, chocolate, fruits and vegetables. The antioxidant effects may play a role in slowing aging, fighting cancer, reducing blood clotting, preventing obesity, relaxing blood vessels and slowing atherosclerosis.

Until recently, most reports of the benefits of green tea were anecdotal or from laboratory models or animal studies. Also, the few clinical studies that were available were from the Far East, and thus confounded by lifestyle factors such as higher consumption of fish and soy protein that could also confer a health benefit. Still, a review of population trials suggested that in patients drinking three or more cups a day of green tea, the rate of MI was 11 percent lower.

Recently published clinical studies controlling for these other variables seem to indicate definite benefits of green tea consumption. A study of 500 Japanese men and women consuming at least four cups of green tea daily showed a reduced risk of CHD in men. In another Japanese study, 240 men and women consuming green tea extract showed lower blood pressure and LDL-C and more weight loss than those not receiving the supplement. A Dutch study of over 3,000 men and women found less atherosclerosis and more weight loss in those participants who reported drinking more green tea. A Greek study demonstrated that drinking green tea improved blood flow in the brachial artery within 30 minutes of consumption and that this effect was due to improved endothelial health.

In addition to the antioxidant effects, green tea has been shown to lower total cholesterol and LDL-C and raise HDL-C. This may be due to reduced intestinal absorption of cholesterol. The average drop in LDL-C has been shown to be between 15 percent and 20 percent, which is about what would occur with a low dose of a low-potency statin. The antioxidant EGCG also mimics the actions of insulin and has been shown to reduce blood sugar levels.

Depending on the brand, two or three cups of green tea will provide between 240 and 320 milligrams of EGCG. Green tea extracts are sold as dried leaf tea in capsule form. Supplements are sold with varying amounts of EGCG content. The recommended daily dosage of the extract is 150–750 milligrams. The caffeine-free variety is recommended. Since the EGCG content is much more predictable, in most cases drinking the green tea rather than using supplements will be the most beneficial. There is no benefit proven in terms of weight loss, cholesterol reduction or CHD risk in comparisons of natural green tea versus the extract found in supplements. In most cases, the natural green tea will also be less expensive.

Green tea extract has been associated with heart arrhythmias, hypertension, kidney and liver disorders and stomach ulcers, mainly due to the caffeine content. Individuals with these conditions or pregnant and breast-feeding women should not consume green tea.

4. Vitamin D (OTC 1,000–5,000 IU/day, $10–25/year; Rx available). Vitamin D deficiency has recently been found to be much more prevalent than previously thought. This may be related to both inadequate dietary intake and limited sun exposure. As medical professionals have promoted the public health benefits of reduced fat intake, there has resulted a reduction in the intake of fat-soluble vitamins A, D, E and K. For vitamin D, this reduction is compounded by the public health emphasis on limiting sun exposure because of the increased risk of skin cancer, which has further caused reduced vitamin D levels in the general population.

Vitamin D is necessary for critical metabolic functions supporting bones, immunity and the cardiovascular system. Vitamin D is, in fact, not a vitamin, but is a hormone that is derived from cholesterol. It is initially made in the skin, altered in the liver, and ultimately made by the kidneys into the active hormone calcitrol, also known as vitamin D_3. Vitamin D regulates bone growth, muscle function and inflammation and also influences over 2,000 genes that regulate cellular differentiation and proliferation.

Until recently, the evidence of beneficial health effects of vitamin D combined with calcium supplementation has been confined to improved bone health and reduced risk of fractures in elderly women. The Institute of Medicine recommends daily vitamin D intake of 600 IU for all individuals less than 70 years of age and 800 IU for those 71 and above.

Recent clinical data suggests cardiovascular benefits from vitamin D also. Vitamin D lowers the level of hormones that regulate blood pressure. It improves insulin resistance, endothelial function, arterial inflammation and vascular tone. Individuals with a deficiency of Vitamin D are 40 percent more likely to have hypertension and 30 percent more likely to have abnormal left ventricular heart function. A recent study of 3,400 older Americans found that compared to people with normal vitamin D levels, those with reduced levels were four times more likely to die from all causes as well as from CHD. A study from the Harvard School of Public Health reported that men with vitamin D deficiency had double the risk of having an MI than men with normal levels. Vitamin D deficiency has also been reported to increase the risk of congestive heart failure (CHF) and stroke. Finally, in patients taking statins, vitamin D supplementation may reduce the risk of statin-related muscle problems.

Vitamin D deficiency can be diagnosed through blood testing for 25-hydroxy vitamin D, the chemical form in which vitamin D is stored in the body. A blood level of 35–40 ng/mL (or 90–100 nmol/L) is considered ideal, and a level of less than 10 ng/mL is considered deficient. The only natural food source of vitamin D is fatty fish like salmon, tuna and sardines. Many juices and cereals have additional vitamin D added (or fortified) to enhance their nutritional value. Thus, there are abundant natural sources of vitamin D.

A recent meta-analysis of nearly 1,500 clinical trials evaluating the effects of vitamin D and calcium supplementation on CHD concluded that while calcium supplements with or without vitamin D do not confer a cardiovascular benefit, vitamin D supplementation alone in moderate to high doses may be beneficial in reducing the risk of CHD. Vitamin D supplementation has been shown to lower systolic blood pressure and the risk of diabetes. In kidney dialysis patients, who are commonly deficient in vitamin D, supplementation cuts the risk of death by one-half. A recent study looking at vitamin D-deficient patients who increased their levels to normal found a 25 percent reduced risk of MI, kidney disease, CHF and death, when compared to patients who maintained low levels of vitamin D. A meta-analysis of all of the controlled trials that looked at the effects of supplementation for all types of patients found that supplementation reduced the risk of CHD mortality by 8 percent. Low vitamin D levels are associated with higher levels of CRP, possibly indicating that vitamin D supplementation may be protective against CHD by reducing arterial inflammation, and that the patients who will derive the most benefit are those with low vitamin D and/or high CRP levels.

Based upon scientific data such as this, many experts believe the Institute of Medicine recommended doses for supplementation are too low. The current data suggests that irrespective of their vitamin D levels, given the risk and prevalence of even mild deficiency in older patients, people over the age of 50 should take 1,000 IU (International Units) of Vitamin D_3 (the active form, calcitrol) per day. If true deficiency is documented based upon blood levels, this amount should be increased under the supervision of a physician. Currently ongoing studies of the effects of supplementation may provide further insight.

There are hazards to too much vitamin D. Blood levels of greater than 50 ng/mL have been associated with a rise in CRP levels, as well as an increased risk of certain types of cancer and heart arrhythmias like atrial fibrillation.

5. Niacin (OTC 500–3,000 mg/day, $100–600/year; Rx available). The B_3 vitamin niacin is available as an OTC supplement as well as a prescription medication. Taking niacin is one of the best ways to raise

HDL-C. Niacin blocks the breakdown of fats in adipose tissue, and so decreases free fatty acids in the bloodstream. This decrease in free fatty acids causes the liver to make less VLDL, LDL and cholesterol. The lowering of VLDL has a reciprocal effect on HDL particles, which are caused to increase. Typically, therapeutic doses of niacin will lower triglycerides by 30 percent and LDL-C by 15 percent and raise HDL-C by 20–30 percent. Other lipid benefits include lowering of Lp(a) by 10–30 percent, reducing Apo B100, as well as reducing the number of atherogenic small, dense LDL particles. When niacin is combined with statin therapy, its favorable lipid effects are even more pronounced. However, the risk of toxicities that accompany the use of statin medications, especially muscle and kidney damage, is also increased.

Scientific data over 30 years has shown multiple benefits from niacin intake. There is substantial evidence that immediate-release niacin reduces the risk of CHD. It has been shown to prevent a first heart attack, to prevent a recurrent heart attack in patients who have already had CHD and to reverse atherosclerosis. A recent meta-analysis of 11 randomized clinical trials of immediate- and extended-release niacin confirmed that niacin reduces the risk of CHD events and the progression of atherosclerosis in nearly all types of patients studied.

A recent clinical trial called the AIM-HIGH trial, published in 2011, has called into question the beneficial effects of extended-release niacin for patients with known CHD who are already on statin therapy. In this study, patients with well-controlled LDL-C levels derived no additional benefit from niacin, despite its effect to increase HDL-C levels. For unexplained reasons, and in numbers not statistically significant, more patients receiving niacin had strokes. Of note, patients assigned to placebo therapy in this study actually received a 50–100 milligram dose of immediate-release niacin. Could the small dose of niacin actually have been protective? As we can see, the use of niacin supplements and prescriptions remains an area of evolving knowledge. Still, it seems reasonable to consider immediate-release niacin supplements if your HDL level is low and you do not have CHD and are also not on statin therapy.

Niacin has several side effects, the most noticeable of which is flushing and itching of the skin. This is caused by the release of a family of chemicals called prostaglandins. These cause the capillaries under the skin to dilate, making the skin tingle, sting and turn red. It is considered a nuisance side effect, rather than a sign of any toxicity of the chemical. With continued use, the itching and flushing resolve. Taking aspirin 30 minutes before taking the niacin will significantly reduce the symptoms, as will taking the niacin with a low-fat snack, avoiding alcohol and taking the niacin before going to bed at night. Niacin can also raise blood sugar, and should be monitored very carefully in diabetics and those individuals with metabolic syndrome.

It is worth noting that, as a supplement, only the immediate-release form of OTC niacin has proven benefits. There are two other forms of nia-cin available in OTC preparations. The non-flush niacin contains inositol esterified with niacin. It has very limited lipid efficacy because very little of the free niacin enters the bloodstream. Sustained-release forms of niacin are also available as OTC supplements. These preparations show extreme vari-ability in how quickly and how much niacin is actually released into the bloodstream. Furthermore, not only have they not been proven to raise HDL-C, they also carry a significant risk of causing liver damage. It is rec-ommended that all niacin preparations be administered under the supervi-sion of a physician. Prescription niacin is available as multiple unbranded immediate release preparations, or the branded extended-release form mar-keted under the name Niaspan. This is discussed along with other prescrip-tion lipid medications in Chapter 13.

"This Stuff Might Work:" Probably Effective and Safe

The compounds in this section have been shown to favorably affect lipids and/or have evidence to support a heart benefit from both anecdotal reports and clinical trials. However, not all studies have found consistent benefits. In some cases, side effects have also been reported that need to be considered when weighing the risks and benefits of using these compounds. There may be other medical benefits beyond those related to the heart for these compounds.

6. Testosterone (OTC, as DHEA, 25–50 mg/day, $100/year; Rx available). Most men experience a normal drop in testosterone levels beginning in their 20s. The decline continues at a fairly rapid pace until the age of 50, at which time testosterone levels stabilize. The symptoms of "male menopause" are thought to be attributable to this decline. It is estimated that low testosterone levels are present in two to four million men in the United States, but only five percent receive treatment. Declining testosterone is linked to loss of muscle mass and strength, gain of abdominal fat, bone loss and cognitive decline. Other signs include slower growth of hair, less need to shave, loss of height, hot flashes, sweats and erectile dysfunction (ED). Up to 20 percent of ED is associated with low testosterone levels.

In addition to fueling the sex drive, testosterone may be protective against CHD, metabolic syndrome and diabetes. Furthermore, the production of testosterone is suppressed by low-fat diets, which are often used in managing CHD risk. This can result in impaired muscle growth and fat burning and actually contribute to an increase in belly fat and central obesity. Low testosterone in men is a risk factor for metabolic syndrome and diabetes. Men with higher testosterone levels are 75 percent less likely to be obese than those with low testosterone levels.

Several studies have shown that low testosterone levels are associated with an increased risk of death of up to 40 percent compared to men who have normal testosterone levels. This risk appeared to be independent of other CHD risk factors like diabetes and obesity. Some studies indicate that men who have heart attacks and strokes often have lower than normal testosterone levels for their age.

Testosterone therapy has been shown to reduce body fat, decrease LDL-C and improve insulin sensitivity. Injections of testosterone in men with congestive heart failure have been shown to improve muscle strength and insulin resistance. In patients with angina, oral testosterone has been shown to relieve anginal symptoms. In laboratory studies, testosterone administration dilates coronary arteries, lowers blood pressure and improves heart function. These observations have fueled an interest in testosterone supplementation in the prevention and treatment of CHD.

Testosterone supplementation is confounded by the fact that testosterone blood tests are complicated and difficult to interpret. Over 97 percent of the testosterone circulating in the blood is bound to blood proteins.

However, it is the amount that circulates unbound that really matters when it comes to signs and symptoms of deficiency. Most blood tests report both total and free testosterone. Further complicating the issue is that testosterone levels vary during the day, with the most production and highest blood level in the morning and the lowest in the evening. There is also significant variation in blood levels within the same individual as well as considerable overlap between age groups that further complicates both diagnosis and treatment.

The diagnosis of testosterone deficiency is made when suspicious symptoms are confirmed by abnormally low blood levels of free testosterone. In such patients, testosterone supplementation under a physician's supervision has shown some benefit. Testosterone supplementation should not be given to men with prostate or breast cancer.

Testosterone is best supplemented in prescription form and under a physician's supervision. One convenient method is a prescription gel that is rubbed on the skin daily. Injections of testosterone can also be given and can be administered weekly, monthly or quarterly. There are also prescription transdermal patches that permit slow absorption through the skin. They can be applied daily, and eliminate the need to manually apply the gel. Transdermal preparations are the most expensive. There are also sublingual forms of testosterone that can be absorbed under the tongue or the cheek.

Oral testosterone is not very effective because in pill form testosterone is quickly metabolized by the liver as soon as it is absorbed through the stomach, by what is known as the "first pass effect." Thus, blood levels remain very low. There are no oral testosterone supplements available in the United States. DHEA (dehydroepiandrosterone) is a steroid hormone that is often marketed as a natural means of testosterone supplementation in oral form. It is a natural chemical made by the adrenal glands. It functions as a precursor to both testosterone and estrogen. DHEA supplements are typically used to combat autoimmune conditions. They have also been reported to boost testosterone levels.

No long-term trials of either oral testosterone supplementation or DHEA have shown significant benefits in blood lipids, diabetes, weight or the risk of CHD events. In fact, there are significant risks associated with testosterone supplementation that make it advisable that it be taken only under medical supervision. These include liver problems, baldness, fluid retention, breast enlargement and an increased risk of prostate cancer. Testosterone supplementation lowers sperm counts and thus should be avoided by men who still want children. Testosterone can raise the amount of red blood cells and make the blood more viscous. Testosterone supplementation has also been shown to lower HDL-C levels, which may actually promote atherosclerosis.

7. Red Yeast Rice (OTC 2,400 mg/day, $250/year). The extract of red yeast rice contains the chemical Monacolin K. This is the same active chemical that is found in the statin lovastatin, or Mevacor. In fact, lovastatin, like some other statins, is termed a "fungal" statin, since the active ingredient is derived from red yeast, which is in fact a fungus. In addition, red yeast rice extract also contains plant sterols, monounsaturated fats and antioxidants that may also assist in its beneficial effects on lipids.

Red yeast rice supplements work in the same way as statins do, by blocking the key enzyme HMG-CoA reductase, in the pathway to the manufacture of cholesterol. They have been shown to lower total cholesterol, LDL-C and triglycerides. The potency of red yeast rice is two to five percent of the potency of the lowest statin dose available, but even at that level it has been shown to lower LDL-C by five–15 percent. However, there are no studies evaluating CHD prevention, treatment and reversal with red yeast rice.

Whether a red yeast rice supplement works or not depends on the formulation. There are many formulations and many brands. Some work, some don't. Since there is no FDA standardization, ultimately, the only way to know the effectiveness of the supplement is to have your baseline cholesterol checked, start taking red yeast rice at the therapeutic dosage of 2,400 milligrams a day, and then recheck your blood lipid panel in two months. If you don't see a change, try a different brand of red yeast rice supplement.

Like statins, red yeast rice can have side effects, such as muscle pain, tenderness and possibly liver damage. Doses higher than 2,400 milligrams per day are not recommended, and if any symptoms of toxicity develop, the supplement should be stopped and a medical evaluation performed. Red yeast rice should not be used in patients taking statin medications or those with liver disease. It may also increase the risk of bleeding and should be used with caution by people taking blood thinners.

"My Neighbor Says This Worked:" Conflicting Data on Efficacy and Safety

The compounds discussed in this section are widely advertised and touted to have heart benefits. There is some evidence to support either a lipid or CHD outcome benefit, but the data is contradicted by other studies showing no benefit. In most cases, the consensus of opinion is that they are not likely of significant benefit unless specific situations exist that would enhance their value, such as deficiency states. They may have other health benefits outside of the heart. There may be risks or side effects associated with their use.

8. **Policosanol (OTC 10–80 mg/day, $100–200/year)**. Policosanol is a natural extract of beeswax and plant waxes, derived primarily from sugarcane and yams. A number of benefits have been ascribed to policosanol, including lowering cholesterol and improving circulation in the legs and heart. It has been shown to have effects similar to statin medications in impairing the production of cholesterol by affecting the enzyme HMG-CoA reductase. Policosanol may also lower cholesterol through inhibiting the absorption of cholesterol-containing bile acids and also by increasing the elimination of LDL-C. Some studies have shown that it can raise HDL-C as well. It may also have antiplatelet properties that make platelets less sticky, and thus reduce the risk of blood clots.

Most of the studies supporting health benefits of policosanol have been conducted or funded in Cuba, where most of the world's policosanol is produced and marketed. A meta-analysis of 52 studies, primarily from Cuba, found that taking policosanol reduced LDL-C by 24 percent, and was more effective than taking plant sterols, which reduced LDL-C by only ten percent. Policosanol also improved total cholesterol, HDL-C, and triglyceride levels more favorably than plant sterols. Studies outside of Cuba, from Germany, Canada and South Africa have not shown the same beneficial results. No study has yet to show a reduced risk of CHD with Policosanol.

One significant concern with policosanol is that it can interact with blood thinners and statins to increase the risk of side effects. Liver problems and muscle tenderness, along with GI symptoms have been reported. Increased bleeding and bruising have also been reported. Thus, policosanol should not be used with statins or blood thinners, including OTC medications like aspirin, ibuprofen and naproxen.

9. Magnesium (OTC 400–800 mg/day, $100–250/year; Rx available). The primary role of magnesium supplementation has been to treat or prevent heart arrhythmias caused by magnesium deficiency. Recent evidence indicates that magnesium may also be of value in the efficient contraction of the heart muscle, with deficiency potentially contributing to congestive heart failure. Magnesium may also play a role in plaque stabilization as well as preventing arterial spasm through its beneficial effect on the arterial endothelium. Finally, magnesium may play a role in lipid regulation, as it has been shown to lower triglycerides.

It is estimated that up to 50 percent of all Americans are magnesium deficient. This is likely related to our preference for processed foods, which are much lower in magnesium than natural foods. In most cases, magnesium deficiency is mild and can easily be corrected by increasing the intake of natural foods high in magnesium. Such foods are prevalent across a variety of classes, some of which include whole-grain breads and cereals, soy beans, lima beans, avocados, spinach, beets, cashews, peanuts and raisins. Magnesium deficiency is especially common and problematic in patients taking diuretics, commonly known as water pills. It is also common in alcoholics. In such patients, or those with persistently low measured levels of magnesium, magnesium supplementation may be of value.

There are large clinical trials that have shown magnesium deficiency is associated with heart disease. An analysis of magnesium levels in over 88,000 women, over 26 years of follow-up in the Nurses' Health Study showed that those women with the highest levels of magnesium were 37 percent less likely to experience the syndrome of sudden cardiac death than those with the lowest levels. The Honolulu Heart Study found patients with the lowest levels of magnesium intake (50–186 milligrams) had twice the risk of MI compared to those with highest intake (340–1,183 milligrams).

The six-year Iowa Women's Health Study of 39,000 patients suggested that chronic magnesium deficiency may promote diabetes.

The evidence to support supplementing magnesium to treat or prevent heart problems is less persuasive. The best trial to date addressing this was a 2003 study of 187 patients with CHD who were followed for six months, and showed that subjects had better exercise tolerance and reduced angina when they received magnesium supplements. Aside from this study, no large-scale clinical trial of magnesium supplementation has been conducted to evaluate the cardiovascular benefits.

There are risks to taking magnesium supplements. Magnesium works as a laxative and is the major ingredient in milk of magnesia. Magnesium can also accumulate to dangerous and toxic levels in patients with kidney problems. Thus, magnesium should be avoided by patients who have chronic kidney disease.

10. Garlic (OTC 400–1,200 mg/day, $40–100/year). Garlic is an herb that has long been touted throughout history to have medicinal effects. Aside from being able to ward off vampires, it has reported value in preventing various types of cancer, prostate problems and a variety of day-to-day illnesses ranging from hay fever to jock itch. Supplements made from the clove of garlic are available for use without a prescription.

The active ingredient in garlic is allicin. This compound is rich in organosulfur chemicals, which give garlic its distinctive pungent smell. Allicin, also found in onions, is a potent antioxidant. Garlic also has a high content of the antioxidant selenium. Garlic can be made odorless by aging the allicin. However, this also reduces its medicinal effectiveness. Thus, some odorless garlic supplements may contain very little of the active ingredient that gives garlic its medicinal benefit.

The beneficial effects of garlic for the heart and circulation have modest scientific support. Garlic has been shown to reduce systolic blood pressure by seven to eight percent in patients who have hypertension. It can also lower blood pressure in patients with normal blood pressure. Garlic may lower LDL-C and reduce platelet stickiness. It may also help boost immunity.

Studies evaluating garlic in the treatment of CHD have yielded conflicting results. The greatest support for a beneficial role for garlic in CHD comes from a 2004 trial looking at coronary artery CAT scans in 21 patients. The results showed that with the addition of garlic supplement in nine patients, plaque advanced by only seven and one-half percent compared to a progression of 22 percent in those who received a placebo. However, most studies have found no significant change in lipid levels among subjects taking garlic supplements, including a large 2007 randomized clinical trial funded by the National Institutes of Health (NIH). A trial in patients with peripheral arterial disease found no change in improved blood flow to the legs after 12 weeks of garlic supplementation.

The variability in the noted health benefits of garlic may well be related to the inconsistency in bioavailability of the active ingredients in supplements. Garlic may cause GI side effects, including heartburn, nausea and diarrhea. It may increase the risk of bleeding and should be taken with extreme care, if at all, by patients using anticoagulant medications or fish oil.

11. CoQ10, or Ubiquinol (OTC 100–200 mg/day, $200–500/year). Coenzyme Q10, or CoQ10, also known as ubiquinol, is a fat-soluble compound that has several purported health benefits. These range from protection from and treatment for age-related neurodegenerative diseases like Parkinson's disease, Alzheimer's disease and Lou Gehrig's disease to retarding the aging process itself to ameliorating circulation disorders.

CoQ10 functions to assist in the transport of electrons used to make ATP (adenosine tri-phosphate), the energy storehouse chemical of our cells that is made by mitochondria. In addition to its value in enhancing energy stores in the heart, CoQ10 also appears to be an antioxidant. It may protect circulating LDL particles from oxidation and incorporation into arterial plaque.

CoQ10 deficiency has been found to be more prevalent in patients with CHD. This appears to be especially true of patients that have weakened or damaged hearts and suffer from CHF. One of the best-studied roles for a heart benefit from CoQ10 has been in patients with CHF. A 1994 study reported that 78 percent of patients with CHF receiving CoQ10 supplements had an improved quality of life. Small studies have shown that it may have a protective effect in patients in the midst of an acute heart attack, and may enhance recovery in patients having heart surgery. It has modest effects in lowering blood pressure and blood sugar. However, no clinical trial has found that CoQ10 supplementation will prevent, treat or reverse CHD.

In patients taking statin drugs for high cholesterol, CoQ10 was shown in a 2005 study to help prevent muscle pains or liver damage that occurs in some people taking statin drugs. The debate on this continues, as other studies have not shown the same benefit. Some researchers believe that statins may block the natural formation of CoQ10 in muscle cells, which could contribute to muscle damage.

12. Acetyl L-Carnitine (OTC 500–3,000 mg/day, $250–500/year). Acetyl L-carnitine is a derivative of the amino acid Lysine. It is found primarily in meat and dairy products, but can also be made by the liver and kidneys. Deficiency of acetyl L-carnitine is exceedingly rare, even among true vegans. Like CoQ10, the amino acid Acetyl L-carnitine is postulated to increase ATP production within heart muscle cells, and so boost cellular energy. It may also have antioxidant effects like CoQ10.

There is no evidence to support the use of acetyl L-carnitine in the prevention of CHD, the treatment of lipid disorders or other CHD risk factors. The benefits of acetyl L-carnitine supplementation in the treatment of CHD patients with angina, CHF patients and patients afflicted with leg pain due to peripheral vascular disease have been reported in small clinical trials. However, in all of these conditions, other studies conducted in similar patients have failed to show a benefit. It should be noted that in all of these trials, acetyl-L-carnitine was added to conventional therapy, not in place of conventional therapy.

The two large-scale, randomized, controlled-clinical trials of acetyl L-carnitine, one in 472 patients, and the other in 2,330 patients, found no short or long-term benefit in treating CHD patients who survived a heart attack. Therefore, the generalized use of acetyl L-carnitine is not advised, although in certain patients with angina, CHF or leg pain due to peripheral vascular disease, and who have not responded well to conventional therapy, there may be a role for acetyl-L-carnitine supplementation. Side effects are primarily GI in nature, and it may increase the risk of seizures in patients with epilepsy.

Antioxidant Vitamins. The antioxidant vitamins C, E and A have been of great interest as potential mediators for preventing and reversing CHD. A number of controlled clinical trials are now available to evaluate their efficacy and safety claims. Most studies have looked at patients either post-MI or patients at high risk for CHD. Some have used synthetic forms of the vitamins, and others have used the natural forms. Dosing in trials was highly variable, with follow-up lasting one to 12 years. Collectively, for the most part, clinical trials have failed to demonstrate a benefit of these antioxidant vitamins in preventing, treating or reversing CHD.

13. Vitamin C (OTC 800–1,000 mg/day, $100/year). The health benefits of vitamin C supplementation have been extensively studied. True vitamin C deficiency is called scurvy and is now only rarely seen in the developed world. At one time it was very prevalent, especially in situations where there was no, or limited, availability of fresh fruit and vegetables, as with sailors on extended voyages. Today, mild degrees of vitamin C deficiency may be found in smokers and elderly patients as well as people under conditions of stress or who use certain medications.

There are a number of postulated heart benefits from vitamin C. It is vital in collagen formation and the structural integrity of many tissues including blood vessels. Its beneficial effects include lowering of blood pressure and improving endothelial function, antioxidant properties and anti-inflammatory effects in arteries, as evidenced by the reduction of CRP levels. Vitamin C has not been found to have a significant impact on blood lipids, but may lower Lp(a), the "heart attack protein" particle that is attached to LDL particles.

Several large and well-designed studies evaluating the heart benefits of vitamin C supplementation have been conducted. The results have been mixed and controversial. The First National Health and Nutrition Examination Survey Epidemiologic Follow-up Study found a reduced risk of CHD events in patients who took vitamin C supplements or had a high dietary intake of vitamin C. The risk of CHD events was decreased by 42 percent in men and by 25 percent in women. Another study of patients who had had angioplasty to treat coronary artery blockages found a 50 percent reduced rate of needing repeat angioplasty in patients who took vitamin C. An Italian study in 2002 looking at progression of plaque over a ten-year period in patients with carotid artery and peripheral arterial disease found reduced plaque progression among those patients receiving vitamin C supplementation. Additionally, the vitamin C group also showed a remarkable 43 percent reduction in mortality.

However, in several larger observational studies, vitamin C supplementation has not been associated with reduced CHD event risk or mortality. In a secondary prevention trial of cholesterol reduction and effect on the development of coronary artery stenosis, vitamin C supplementation was of no benefit. Finally, no primary prevention trial of vitamin C supplementation has shown that vitamin C prevents the development of CHD.

One reason that supplementation may not be as effective as increasing dietary intake is that vitamin C may work better when combined with the super antioxidant compounds known as bioflavanoids. Most fruits and vegetables contain both vitamin C and bioflavanoids together. However, as a supplement, these compounds are often stripped away from vitamin C. As a supplement, the esterified form is better absorbed but is also more expensive. Side effects of vitamin C include the development of stomach ulcers and acid reflux, as vitamin C is the chemical ascorbic acid. Consuming more than 200 milligrams daily of vitamin C has been shown to inhibit the anti-inflammatory effects of statins. Therefore, vitamin C should not be used in patients taking statin medications.

14. Vitamin E or D-Alpha Tocopherol (OTC vitamin E 400 IU/day, d-alpha tocopherol 15 mg/day, both $150/year). The natural form of vitamin E, d-alpha tocopherol, is an antioxidant with reported health benefits. Consuming large amounts of vitamin E has been shown to reduce the risk of Alzheimer's disease. It has also been shown to reduce the risk of dying from the neurodegenerative disease amyotrophic lateral sclerosis (ALS, Lou Gehrig's disease). Natural sources of vitamin E are nuts or seeds, green leafy vegetables, legumes, papaya, whole grains, soybean, sweet potatoes and watercress. Since it is not water soluble, it is not commonly found in most fruits and vegetables.

The evidence supporting a beneficial role for vitamin E in CHD is controversial. The greatest support for preventing CHD comes from both the Nurses' Health Study in women and the Health Professionals study in men, which found a reduced risk of CHD events by 37 and 25 percent, respectively. However, if the participants took vitamin E for short periods of time (less than 2–4 years), or at doses of less than 100 IU, no risk reduction was noted. In the treatment of patients who already have CHD, the

Cambridge Heart Antioxidant Study (CHAOS) found a reduced risk of CHD events after one and one-half years of vitamin E supplementation.

Counter to these trials are multiple trials that have failed to show a benefit of vitamin E in preventing or treating CHD. Both the Iowa Women's Health Study and Physician's Health Study found no prevention benefit of vitamin E supplementation. A trial specifically designed to look at the question, called the Alpha-Tocopherol Beta-Carotene (ATBC) study also found no prevention benefit. Furthermore, in this trial, patients with known CHD also experienced no treatment benefit with respect to improvement in angina, CHD events or mortality. Similarly, the Heart Outcomes and Prevention Evaluation (HOPE) trial, which was primarily designed to evaluate the effectiveness of the category of blood pressure medications known as angiotensin converting enzyme inhibitors in patients at high risk for CHD, found no risk reduction of CHD events when 400 IU of vitamin E was administered. Finally, the GISSI-P trial of over 11,000 men and women in Italy, which showed a substantial benefit to omega-3 fish oil supplementation, found no benefit to vitamin E supplements in reducing the risk of CHD events or mortality.

Given the variable results from the many clinical trials, and the widespread use of vitamin E supplements, the Cleveland Clinic performed a meta-analysis of all of the clinical trials relating to vitamin E supplementation. Their review of more than 80,000 patients studied concluded that vitamin E provided neither a prevention nor treatment benefit for CHD.

Vitamin E supplementation has been reported to have some adverse effects. Some studies like the Women's Angiographic Vitamin and Estrogen (WAVE) Study, as well as the HDL-Atherosclerosis Treatment Study (HATS), showed vitamin E supplements enhanced progression of plaque and increased mortality. In these trials vitamin E also appeared to reduce the efficacy of statin therapy to favorably affect blood lipids and reduce arterial inflammation. Thus, as is the case for vitamin C, vitamin E supplements should also be avoided by patients taking statin medications.

15. Vitamin A or Beta-Carotene (OTC vitamin A 2,500–10,000 IU/day, $10/year; beta-carotene 25,000 IU or 15mg/day, both $15/year). Vitamin A and beta-carotene are not one and the same. Beta-carotene is a precursor to vitamin A. Beta-carotene is prevalent in fruits and vegetables containing carotenoids. Carrots are the best-known source of carotenoids, but these compounds are found in most dark orange, red, and green fruits and vegetables. Once eaten and absorbed in the small intestine, beta-carotene is converted to vitamin A. This is the primary source of dietary vitamin A. To obtain vitamin A directly in our diet requires the ingestion of dairy fats, like butter, or eggs, since it is a fat-soluble vitamin. Large quantities of vitamin A would require ingestion of considerable amounts of saturated dairy fat. Thus, while the body needs vitamin A, it is best obtained dietarily in the form of beta-carotene.

Vitamin A is necessary for a number of metabolic functions, but its primary biological role is in the eye to facilitate vision, particularly dim light vision. It is also a necessary cofactor in DNA replication, thus essential to cell growth and division. Deficiencies of vitamin A are most apparent first in rapidly dividing cells of the skin, scalp, bone marrow and lining of the stomach. This accounts for why poor skin quality, brittle hair, anemia and nausea are frequent signs of vitamin A deficiency. It is important for the maintenance of bone integrity, and deficiency can cause bone loss and bone fractures.

With respect to atherosclerosis, it is its role as an antioxidant that has drawn interest. There is considerable scientific data evaluating the cardiac effects of vitamin A and beta-carotene supplementation. The data strongly indicates not only that there is no significant benefit, but there may be risks associated with supplementation of vitamin A and beta-carotene.

Many of the same trials looking at vitamin C and E also evaluated the value of vitamin A supplements in CHD. There are few trials that support a beneficial effect of vitamin A. The Iowa Women's Health Study found that beta-carotene supplementation over four years of treatment had no significant effect on rates of MI, other CHD events or death rates. Similar results were found in the all-male Physician's Health Study. The ATBC study found healthy individuals receiving beta-carotene supplementation (20 milligrams a day) experienced no beneficial effects on the occurrence of MI, angina, major CHD events or death rates after five to eight years of follow-up. In fact, death from all causes was significantly increased by eight percent with beta-carotene, principally because of increased rates of ischemic heart disease and lung cancer.

Trials in patients with known CHD have also been disappointing. In a group of patients in the ATBC trial with known angina, beta-carotene supplementation did not prevent worsening of angina, major CHD events or death. In a subgroup of patients with a history of prior MI in this study, the incidence of fatal CHD events was in fact, significantly increased with beta-carotene.

The previously referenced meta-analysis study by the Cleveland Clinic regarding vitamin E also looked at the evidence in support of vitamin A as protection against atherosclerosis. The researchers pooled results from large randomized trials of beta-carotene use in 138,113 patients. Their results showed that beta-carotene supplementation led to small but statistically significant increase in mortality from any cause, and a slight increase in death due to CHD events.

Thus, the consensus is that Vitamin A and beta-carotene are best obtained naturally from fruits and vegetables that contain carotenoids. Supplementation should be reserved for those individuals with documented deficiency or certain patients with specific visual problems. The use of supplements provides no cardiovascular benefit, and may in fact increase the risk of death and CHD events.

Multivitamin A, C and E Combination Antioxidants. Proponents of antioxidant vitamin therapy for CHD point out that single vitamin supplementation may not be sufficient to demonstrate benefit and that antioxidant therapies work best when multiple antioxidants are combined. A number of clinical trials have addressed this concern. The Heart Protection Study (HPS) looked at more than 20,000 subjects without known CHD in a trial of a combination supplement of vitamin C, vitamin E and beta-carotene. Data on cardiovascular events, vascular mortality and all-cause mortality were collected. The antioxidant supplement group and the placebo group did not differ in rates of mortality, CHD events or need for coronary revascularization.

Several studies of antioxidant vitamin supplementation for prevention of CHD events in patients already diagnosed with CHD have also been conducted. In the Multivitamins and Probucol (MVP) Study, investigators tested an antioxidant and lipid medication (probucol), an antioxidant vitamin supplement (vitamin C, vitamin E and beta-carotene) and a placebo in patients having had coronary artery angioplasty. This study found that the rate of restenosis in the antioxidant-only group did not differ from that in the placebo group. A similar trial in patients having had coronary angioplasty examined the effects of treatment with the statin Simvastatin compared to antioxidant vitamins (vitamin C, vitamin E, natural beta-carotene and selenium) or placebo. Once again, antioxidant therapy did not significantly affect the rate of restenosis or CHD events three years later.

B-Complex Vitamins: 16. Folic Acid, Folate or Vitamin B_9 (OTC 400–1,000 mcg/day, \$20–40/year); 17. Vitamin B_6 (OTC 40–100 mg/day, \$20–40/year); 18. Vitamin B_{12} (OTC 800–1,000 mcg/day, \$20/year). Elevated levels of the amino acid homocysteine have been associated with CHD. Homocysteine has been found to accelerate atherosclerosis by causing endothelial dysfunction. It may also promote thrombosis. Also, homocysteine levels rise with age and may play a role in the increased risk of CHD in older patients as well as heavy drinkers of alcohol. Rarely, inherited genetic disorders can also cause elevations of homocysteine. Normal levels of homocysteine are typically 10–12 umol/L (micromoles/L), with an elevated state defined by levels that exceed 20 umol/L.

Homocysteine metabolism depends on the interaction of three B-complex vitamins; B_9 or folate, B_6 and B_{12}. A deficiency of these vitamins will result in a rise in homocysteine levels. Supplementation with these vitamins will restore normal homocysteine levels. Of these three B vitamins, folate is the least available in the typical American diet. It is found in fruits and vegetables, but only 24 percent of Americans eat the recommended minimum amount of two servings per day.

In the 1950s and 1960s research emerged showing that spinal cord and neurological defects in babies were associated with folate deficiency. As a result, in 1998 the U.S. FDA mandated supplementation of folic acid in all grains, cereals, rice, pasta and breads. Folate refers to the naturally occurring form of vitamin B_9, whereas folic acid is the synthetic form of the vitamin.

Several studies support the use of folic acid supplementation in treating and preventing CHD. In a study of 205 patients undergoing coronary angioplasty, there was a reduced risk of restenosis and CHD events when the patients were given folate, B_6 and B_{12} supplements. The HOPE-2 trial in 2006 reported a reduced risk of stroke in patients receiving B-complex vitamin supplements, although overall death rates were not changed.

The majority of supportive studies have been either anecdotal or with small numbers of patients. The routine supplementation with these B vitamins has recently been called into question as a result of a 2008 study of more than 5,000 women at high risk for CHD that showed that daily folic acid, vitamin B_6 and vitamin B_{12} supplementation did not reduce the risk of CHD events, despite lowering the levels of homocysteine. A recent Norwegian study of heart attack survivors with poor heart function also failed to show a benefit of B-complex vitamin supplementation. Most recently, an Australian study following patients with a recent stroke or TIA for two years found no change in the incidence of repeat events in patients who received B-complex vitamin supplements compared to those who did not, despite a reduction in homocysteine levels in those who received the B-complex vitamins. Most significantly, a recent expert consensus panel concluded that elevated homocysteine levels have no meaningful effect on the risk of developing CHD.

Thus, routine B-complex vitamin supplementation is not recommended to prevent CHD or to treat patients with CHD. However, since B-complex vitamin supplementation offers no perceptible risks, it would seem reasonable to offer B-complex vitamin supplements only to patients with elevated homocysteine levels and a history of CHD events.

"Miracle Elixirs and Snake Oil:" No Value and Possibly Risky

These groups of compounds have only limited scientific support for a heart benefit. In general, they should not be used for any cardiovascular purpose, although they may have other health benefits. In some cases, these compounds and treatments may be associated with a significant potential for harm.

19. Vitamin B5, or Pantothenic Acid (OTC 300–900 mg/day, $50–100/year). Pantothenic acid is also a B vitamin but is not involved in homocysteine metabolism. It is used in the synthesis of the energy-generating compound coenzyme A (CoA). Fortunately, vitamin B5 is very prevalent in nearly all foods, and deficiency is very rare. In fact, the name pantothenic acid comes from the Greek word *pantothen*, meaning "from everywhere."

Recall that the enzyme HMG-CoA reductase is a critical component in the pathway of cholesterol synthesis. CoA is also used in fatty acid synthesis. By virtue of these effects, a deficiency of vitamin B_5 has been proposed to result in diminished synthesis of CoA, and thus cause elevations of total cholesterol, LDL-C, triglycerides and a depression of HDL-C.

Even though vitamin B_5 is exceedingly prevalent, a nutritional supplement is available for use. Several studies in animals in which vitamin B_5 was administered showed reduced total cholesterol, LDL-C and triglyceride levels. Anecdotal studies in human subjects have shown modest benefits in lipids. However, there have been no controlled clinical trials in humans that have shown a benefit of vitamin B_5 supplementation in outcomes to prevent, treat or reverse CHD.

20. L-Lysine (OTC 1,000 mg/day, $250/year). The chemist Dr. Linus Pauling, renowned for promoting the widespread use of vitamin C is also credited with the initial reports of the value of using the amino acid L-Lysine to relieve angina and lower blood pressure. Studies in laboratory models and animals found evidence that lysine may help treat atherosclerosis. A 2007 study from California found that lysine inhibited the biological response of muscle cells lining the arteries to form plaque in laboratory models. It is based upon this data that L-Lysine is promoted as a supplement to relieve angina, reduce blood pressure, and treat CHD. There are no clinical trials in human subjects that attest to either beneficial treatment or prevention benefits of lysine for atherosclerosis or CHD.

Lysine may cause GI distress, and individuals with liver or kidney disease should avoid taking lysine, as aggravation of preexisting conditions in these organs has been reported.

21. L-Arginine (OTC 6–9 gm/day, $200/year). L-arginine is an amino acid that is important in the regulation of arterial blood flow. L-arginine is a precursor to the formation of nitric oxide, a compound known to cause arterial relaxation through its actions on the endothelium. Because of this action, it has been postulated that L-arginine's benefits might be to lower blood pressure, improve circulation and even help with erectile dysfunction.

Deficiencies of L-arginine are rare. It is abundant in many different types of foods, including red meat, fish, poultry, wheat germ, chocolate, grains, nuts, seeds and dairy products. The body also has the capability to synthesize it from other amino acids.

Data supporting the cardiovascular benefits of L-arginine supplementation is sparse. There are anecdotal reports that it may reduce angina. A 2006 Johns Hopkins study of 153 patients found L-arginine supplementation had no effect on arterial stiffness, heart function, symptoms of CHD or CHD outcomes. There are no long-term studies of L-arginine evaluating CHD or lipid benefits.

There are minor side effects to L-arginine supplementation, including GI symptoms, gout and worsening of asthma. It was found to increase the mortality rate in patients following an MI, and therefore should not be used in such patients.

22. D-Ribose (OTC 5–15 gm/day, $250–500/year). Like CoQ10 and L-carnitine, D-ribose is also a chemical that plays a role in energy metabolism. It is found in abundance in red meat. It is postulated that normally functioning heart muscle cells can generate enough D-ribose to function properly, but that damaged or stressed cells may become deficient, so that supplementation may be necessary.

Improved blood pressure and exercise capacity in CHF patients has been noted. D-ribose may lower blood sugar. Clinical data supporting a beneficial role for D-ribose in preventing, treating or reversing CHD does not exist. Aside from minor GI symptoms as well as mild hypoglycemia, no significant toxicities to consumption of D-ribose have been reported.

23. Resveratrol (OTC 100–500 mg/day, $250–500/year). There is experimental evidence in animals to indicate that the chemical resveratrol may reduce cholesterol and blood sugar, slow aging, and reduce inflammation, oxidation and blood clotting. Resveratrol is found naturally in red wine, grapes, and other fruits. Statistical data in individuals who consume such foods containing resveratrol suggests that these individuals have a reduced risk of CHD. Based upon such evidence, this supplement has been promoted to be beneficial in preventing and treating CHD.

Resveratrol is available as a supplement in the form of either grapeseed extract or from the Japanese knotweed. As a result of extensive news coverage, sales of resveratrol supplements increased dramatically in the years 2004–2006. Nevertheless, the clinical benefits of resveratrol by itself are largely unfounded.

Resveratrol is an antioxidant. It has been speculated that it confers some of the health benefit attributed uniquely to red wine, since it is found in grape skins. However, to get the health benefits of resveratrol at the doses that were demonstrated in animal studies, an individual would have to consume the equivalent of 60 liters of red wine per day. A single glass of red wine contains about one milligram of resveratrol. Oral supplements vary widely in their purity and bioavailability of resveratrol. Furthermore, the majority of orally ingested resveratrol is inactivated by intestinal and liver enzymes before it ever enters the systemic blood circulation.

There are no clinical studies that support the use of resveratrol supplements for any cardiac or health benefit. Side effects can include diarrhea, and liver toxicity has been reported. Thus, if there are cardiovascular benefits of resveratrol, they appear to require that the chemical be ingested as it is packaged in nature, with red wine, grapes or fruits, and not as a stand-alone supplement.

24. Calcium (OTC 1,000–1,600 mg/day, $20/year; Rx available). Calcium supplements, with or without vitamin D, are widely used for the prevention and treatment of osteoporosis. Studies evaluating the benefits of calcium supplementation for heart disease have yielded conflicting results. Studies showing a benefit have suggested that individuals over the age of 50 should take at least 1,000 milligrams per day, and that women should take 1,600 milligrams per day.

A recent re-analysis of data collected in 36,000 patients over a seven year follow-up in the Women's Health Initiative (WHI) study reviewed the effects of calcium supplementation on the risk of CHD events in postmenopausal women. Patients taking prescribed or over the counter calcium supplements had a 13–22 percent higher risk of CHD events than those not taking calcium. When data from other smaller studies is pooled with the WHI data, the use of calcium supplements is associated with a consistent and reproducible increase in the risk of stroke and CHD events by 15 percent and 25 percent, respectively. Even when the benefits for osteoporosis are taken into account, routine calcium supplementation does not provide a net benefit.

Alert! Data from a meta-analysis indicates that routine calcium supplementation in 1,000 women would prevent three bone fractures but would come at a cost of six additional strokes and heart attacks.

A recent re-analysis of the WHI study by investigators from New Zealand, published in 2011 in the *British Medical Journal*, found that calcium supplementation in combination with vitamin D further increased the risk of CHD events and stroke. Calcium in the bloodstream is associated with an increase in carotid plaque and calcium buildup on the aortic valve, as well as an increase in rates of MI and death due to CHD. Calcium may affect the process of plaque formation and may also increase the coaguability of the blood. Both can affect the risk of atherosclerosis as well as events like stroke and heart attack that are also dependent on arterial clot formation.

These data suggest that the routine use of calcium supplements, with or without vitamin D should be discouraged. Calcium supplements may also have other side effects related primarily to the GI system or increasing the risk of kidney stones.

25. Selenium (OTC 200 mcg/day, $15/year). Selenium is a trace mineral with antioxidant properties that may retard atherosclerosis. Some population studies have found lower selenium levels in patients with CHD, compared to patients without CHD. Selenium is found in abundance in many types of plant and animal products and true selenium deficiency is exceedingly rare. Nevertheless, selenium supplements have been promoted as a way to reduce the risk of CHD.

A meta-analysis published in 2006 of 25 small studies conducted between the years 1966–2006 reported that a 50 percent increase in selenium concentration corresponded to a 24 percent decline in the risk of CHD events. However, this same meta-analysis reviewed several small trials in which selenium supplementation was given to individuals at risk for CHD, and found no significant beneficial effect of selenium in preventing CHD. Thus, the data in support of selenium to reduce the risk of CHD has been confusing and inconclusive.

The answer became somewhat clearer with the results of a randomized trial that was published in 2006 from the State University of New York in Buffalo of 1,300 patients receiving selenium supplements over a seven year period. The study reported that selenium supplementation at a dose of 200 mcg/day produced no reduction in the risk of CHD events. Selenium supplements can cause GI side effects, hair loss and nerve damage. Based upon the existing data, selenium supplements are not recommended for cardiovascular disease prevention or treatment.

26. Pomegranate Juice (OTC 250 mg, $70/year; juice 1.5–8 oz/day, $300–800/year). Pomegranates have a very high content of antioxidants, similar to those in red wine, which may retard atherosclerosis. These same chemicals also increase nitric oxide production, which causes blood vessel dilation, reduces endothelial stress and reduces blood pressure. For these reasons, pomegranate juice has been touted as having benefits in preventing and treating CHD.

The evidence supporting a benefit in CHD comes primarily from a three-year Israeli study in which patients with CHD consuming pomegranate juice showed reduced levels of oxidized LDL, blood pressure and evidence of reduced atherosclerosis as assessed by carotid intimal medial thickness (cIMT). The level of carotid plaque was reduced by 35 percent in subjects consuming pomegranate juice, compared to a nine percent increase in control subjects. A criticism of the study was that it included only ten patients.

A follow-up study by the same Israeli investigators in patients without diagnosed CHD showed no overall benefit. Other studies in both patients with and without CHD have shown no consistent benefit in terms of CHD outcomes, blood pressure or lipid levels.

Pomegranate juice has been reported to cause lowering of blood pressure and allergic reactions. Product standardization is also a concern, as some products labeled as 100 percent pomegranate juice have been found to be of inconsistent quality. In 2010, the Federal Trade Commission (FTC) issued an administrative order charging the makers of one brand of pomegranate juice and supplements with making false and unsubstantiated claims stating that their products would prevent or treat heart disease, prostate cancer or erectile dysfunction.

Although pomegranate juice is not likely to cause significant harm for most people, it should be avoided by those with low blood pressure as well as by diabetics because of its sugar content. There is no conclusive evidence that it will provide any significant health benefits, including in the prevention, treatment and reversal of CHD.

27. Acai (OTC 1,000 mg/day, $60/year; juice 2 oz/day, $400/year). The acai berry is a fruit similar to a blueberry that grows on the acai palm tree, which is native to the rainforests of Central and South America. It has been called an "elite superfood" as it has wide ranging purported health benefits including weight loss, anti-aging and as a beauty aid in cosmetics to name just a few. Laboratory studies indicate that it may have antioxidant activity, and like red wine, may therefore help retard atherosclerosis.

The acai juice is the form in which the supplement is most commonly consumed. The antioxidant potency of acai dissipates very quickly once the berry is harvested, processed and stored. It is an excellent source of fiber and plant sterols, and it is likely that the few heart benefits reported may be from this property, rather than as an antioxidant. There do not appear to be any serious side effects of consuming acai. There are no clinical trials that have indicated acai has any notable CHD benefits for prevention or treatment.

28. Noni (OTC 400 mg/day, $45/year; juice 1 oz/day, $200/year). Noni juice has recently been promoted as possibly having health benefits specifically related to lowering blood lipids. The juice derives from the fruit of a Polynesian plant and is widely available commercially.

The best evidence of a benefit comes from a 2006 study in 106 smokers consuming one to four ounces of noni juice every day for one month, which found reductions of 20–25 percent in total cholesterol and triglycerides. However, the study was funded by the makers of the product, and the product consumed was a mixture of juices of the noni plant as well as blueberries and grapes. Aside from this study, there are no other studies that have reported any benefits on blood lipids. There are no studies that have examined event rates for CHD or other heart benefits of noni juice.

Noni juice is high in potassium and can be dangerous to people with kidney disease. There have also been published case reports of patients who suffered liver damage while consuming noni juice.

29. Lecithin, or Phospholipids/Phosphatidylcholine (OTC 1,500–2,500 mg/day, $500/year). Phosphatidylcholine is a molecule that helps make the fat-soluble cholesterol molecule more water soluble. In the body, phosphatidylcholine is found primarily in cell membranes, and assists in transporting cholesterol within the cell. The major source of dietary choline is from the compound lecithin.

Lecithin and phosphatidylcholine are touted as "fat emulsifiers." The theory suggests that when lecithin is in the bloodstream, it promotes the solubility and movement of cholesterol and fats, thereby preventing these substances from sticking to artery walls. By inhibiting the accumulation of cholesterol against artery walls, lecithin helps maintain a healthy cardiovascular system. Other blood lipid benefits ascribed to lecithin include lowering total cholesterol and LDL-C and promoting reverse cholesterol transport through its effect on either raising HDL-C or making the HDL particle a more effective cholesterol scavenger.

Lecithin is a fat found in egg yolk, liver, peanuts, cauliflower, wheat germ, milk and soybeans. It is also available as an oral supplement, marketed as lecithin, phosphatidylcholine or essential phospholipids. An intravenous form is used in chelation therapy. When used in chelation treatments, it is very expensive, costing up to $150 per treatment. It may also be hazardous in patients with chronic kidney disease.

Early animal experiments suggested that lecithin reduced atherosclerotic plaque, and some anecdotal reports in humans have indicated that it may lessen angina and improve leg circulation. However, there is little or no evidence in any well-controlled clinical trial that supports a cardiovascular benefit of using lecithin or phosphatidylcholine supplements.

30. Chelation (multiple OTC compounds at varying doses, or IV therapy, $600–3,000/year). In traditional chelation therapy, a solution containing chemicals that bind heavy metals is administered to assist in removal of these metals. Chelation therapy has proven value in treating heavy metal intoxication with lead, arsenic or mercury. Aside from this use, there is sparse clinical data to support its use for any other health benefits.

The primary mechanism of benefit in using chelation for treating atherosclerosis is that by binding calcium in the bloodstream, chelation makes less calcium available to enter into atherosclerotic plaque. Since calcium is an integral component of many atherosclerotic plaques, by limiting calcium uptake, plaque will not grow, and may in fact regress. Chelation has been used for all types of atherosclerosis, including the treatment of CHD, stroke and peripheral vascular disease.

Chelation therapy is among the most commonly used "alternative" therapies for CHD. As it is not FDA approved, and its costs are not covered by most insurance plans, it is estimated that CHD patients spend between $400 million and $3 billion annually in out-of-pocket costs for such treatments. It is believed that over 100,000 adults in the U.S. undergo chelation therapy annually for CHD, or about one-quarter the number that undergo CABG surgery.

The most commonly used chelating agent is EDTA (ethylene-diamine-tetra-acetic acid). The intravenous treatments require 30 or more sessions. Patients sit in a chair for several hours receiving the infusions, similar to kidney dialysis. Chelation treatments for CHD can also be performed using orally administered chelating agents that include EDTA among others. The use of Lecithin/phosphatidylcholine is considered a form of oral chelation.

Several controlled clinical trials in relatively small numbers of patients in the 1990s reported that up to 80 percent of patients with CHD had improved symptoms after receiving chelation therapy. Subsequent larger and better designed studies failed to show a benefit. A 2005 systematic review of all published studies evaluating the benefits of chelation therapy in CHD concluded there was no demonstrable benefit to chelation therapy.

To further address the question, a five-year clinical trial evaluating the safety and efficacy of chelation therapy was initiated by the NIH and the U.S. National Center for Complementary and Alternative Medicine in 2003. The trial was suspended in 2008 because of ethical concerns about study subjects receiving appropriate informed consent to participate in the trial. Although near completion at the time it was halted, the trial has never reported any study results. At present, the trial is on the NHLBI list of trials that are "… ongoing, but not recruiting participants." It is unclear if study results will ever be reported.

The FDA, NIH, AHA and the American College of Cardiology have all publicly stated that there is no scientific evidence to support any benefit of chelation therapy in the treatment or prevention of cardiovascular disease. Chelation therapy is associated with side effects, the most serious of which is kidney damage. However, the main concern of chelation is that patients pursuing a route of chelation therapy may be putting themselves at risk by using chelation *in lieu* of accepted treatments for CHD such as life-style modifications, medications, stents and surgery.

Chapter 13
Drug Therapy: Take Two Aspirin and Call Me …

THERE ARE A number of prescription medications that are used in the management of patients who either have or are at risk for developing CHD (coronary heart disease). The approval of medications by the FDA for this purpose is generally predicated upon sound clinical data, typically from controlled clinical trials. However, it is still left to the discretion of each individual health care provider as to exactly how those medications are used in a given patient.

In the management of CHD, the use of medications can be broadly categorized in terms of treatment or prevention. Preventing the development of CHD in at-risk patients is termed primary prevention. Usually these patients have CHD risk factors but no evidence of CHD by signs, symptoms or diagnostic testing. There are an estimated 100 million adults in the United States that are considered patients who are eligible for primary prevention strategies. In all cases, primary prevention strategies start with TLC (therapeutic lifestyle changes) measures, as discussed in Chapters 10 and 11.

The treatment of patients who already have CHD is called secondary prevention. These patients already carry a diagnosis of CHD based upon signs, symptoms, previous CHD events, such as MI, stroke, peripheral vascular disease (PVD), or thoracic or abdominal aortic aneurysms (TAA or AAA), or having had procedures to treat CHD, such as angioplasty, stenting or bypass surgery. Patients without signs, symptoms, previous events or procedures can also be classified as CHD patients based upon testing that indicates they have asymptomatic CHD. There are an estimated 17 million patients in the United States that qualify for secondary prevention.

One very aggressive form of secondary prevention is called CHD reversal. In this case, treatment is aimed not just to prevent future CHD events, but is actually designed to reverse existing atherosclerosis and thus not only reduce the risk of future events but bring the patient back to a lower risk level. Clinical studies evaluating benefits of reversal have directly examined changes in the level of plaque within the artery.

In this chapter, we will discuss the accepted and validated forms of pharmaceutical intervention that have been found to be useful in primary prevention, secondary prevention and reversal of CHD. In general, the medications known to do this can be grouped into two broad categories based upon the mechanism of atherosclerosis that is affected. One form of therapy is directed at the level of the artery. These medications target the arterial processes of endothelial dysfunction, lipid oxidation and/or other plaque growth processes in the arterial wall, and arterial thrombosis. The second grouping is lipid therapy, which primarily targets modifying lipid particles to create a less atherogenic state. In most cases, medications will have several anti-atherosclerotic effects.

Arterial Pharmacotherapy

Beta-Blockers. The class of drugs known as beta-blockers works through reducing the cardiovascular effects of sympathetic nervous system hormones likes adrenaline. In the cardiovascular system, the primary type of beta-receptor is known as the beta-1 receptor, and when stimulated by adrenaline it produces an elevated pulse rate and promotes constriction of the artery and subsequent elevation in blood pressure. By blocking the stimulation of the beta-receptors, the beta-blockers reduce heart rate and blood pressure.

They also prevent some of the other indirect adverse effects of too much sympathetic nervous system stimulation. Through this mechanism, beta-blockers protect the heart from dangerous arrhythmias like atrial fibrillation and ventricular premature beats as well as the more serious and potentially lethal arrhythmias like ventricular tachycardia and ventricular fibrillation. They reduce the workload of the left ventricle, making it work more efficiently and consume less oxygen.

Multiple clinical studies, the largest of which was the Beta-blocker Heart Attack Trial (BHAT) of 4,000 patients followed for two years, have proven that, when used for secondary prevention, beta-blockers reduce the risk of a second MI by up to 50 percent and reduce the risk of death after an MI by 25 percent. Many studies, the most notable of which was the CAPRICORN trial (Carvedilol Post-Infarct Survival Control in Left Ventricular Dysfunction) of nearly 2,000 patients, have shown that beta-blockers prolong survival and improve the quality of life in patients with CHF or with a reduced left ventricular ejection fraction (EF) of less than 40 percent.

Beta-blockers reduce angina symptoms as they improve the balance of coronary artery oxygen supply and demand in patients with CHD. A review of over 4,000 patients with CHD, but without MI or CHF, showed benefit from beta-blocker therapy with a 34 percent reduced chance of death after three years. Thus, because of the overwhelming evidence of benefits, it is recommended that all patients after an MI, and those who have a history of CHF and/or a reduced EF, be on beta-blocker therapy indefinitely. Most patients with angina or CHD will also benefit from beta-blocker therapy.

> **Alert!** One of the biggest problems with use of beta-blockers is that they are underutilized. Surveys consistently show that only 30–50 percent of patients who should be on beta-blockers actually receive them.

For primary prevention of CHD, other than as blood pressure agents, beta-blockers are not of proven value. Thus, unless patients at risk for CHD have need for blood pressure reduction, or need beta-blockers for other symptoms, they are not used in primary prevention.

Beta-blockers can cause fatigue and mental sluggishness. In men, some beta-blockers may cause erectile dysfunction. They may trigger asthma in susceptible individuals or those with chronic lung diseases like emphysema. They can worsen diabetes and in some patients also contribute to depression.

Some of the most common beta-blockers are acebutalol (Sectral), atenolol (Tenormin), carvedilol (Coreg), metoprolol tartrate (Lopressor), metoprolol succinate (Toprol XL), nadolol (Corgard), nebivolol (Bystolic) and propranolol (Inderal).

Anti-Anginal Medications. Angina occurs when oxygen supply and demand are out of balance. While most cases of angina occur due to reduced oxygen supply to the heart caused by coronary plaque obstructions, angina can also occur without the presence of significant blockages. In the latter situation, one cause can be a temporary "spasm" of the coronary artery that temporarily reduces the oxygen supply to the heart. This condition is often termed variant angina, vasospastic angina or Prinzmetal's angina. Another cause of angina without an obstructing level of coronary plaque is when there is an increased demand for oxygen that outstrips the available supply of blood. This is often termed microvascular angina or subendocardial ischemia, as it reflects an inability of the smaller feeder blood vessels that penetrate into the heart muscle to keep up with the oxygen needs of the heart.

While beta-blockers treat angina by reducing the workload of the heart, there are additional medications to treat angina that work by other mechanisms. These medications can be used alongside beta-blockers or as an alternative to beta-blockers. One category of such medications that improve the oxygen supply to the heart is nitrates. Nitrates cause the coronary arteries to dilate, thus improving blood supply and reducing stress on the left ventricle. In fact, immediately putting a rapidly dissolving nitroglycerin tablet or aerosolized spray under the tongue is an extremely effective way to relieve angina and temporarily improve coronary blood supply. Nitrates are available in the rapidly acting aerosolized spray and sublingual dissolving tablets, as well as longer-acting pills and skin patches. Although effective in relieving symptoms, nitrates have not been shown to reduce the chances of future heart attacks or even prevent an ongoing heart attack.

Newer medications have also become available to treat angina. Calcium channel blockers work to both reduce myocardial oxygen demand and improve myocardial oxygen supply. They are not as effective as either beta-blockers or nitrates in either respect, but often offer an excellent compromise to provide both types of beneficial effects over a modest range. Some of the commonly used calcium channel blockers are amlodipine (Norvasc), diltiazem (Cardizem, Tiazac), nifedipine (Procardia, Adalat) and verapamil (Calan, Verelan, Isoptin).

Ranazoline (Ranexa) is an anti-anginal drug that has proved valuable in treating angina, especially in patients who do not respond to the conventional therapies. Ranexa works by blocking what is called the "late sodium channel" in heart cells that are suffering from ischemia. Blocking this sodium channel improves metabolism in ischemic heart cells, reducing damage to the heart muscle and reducing angina symptoms. Neither calcium channel blockers nor Ranazoline have been found to be of benefit in either primary or secondary prevention.

RAAS Blockers. The RAAS blockers are so called because their effects are in the renin-angiotensin-aldosterone system, hence the name RAAS. This is an axis of hormones that originates in the kidney and adrenal gland and serves as the primary regulating mechanism for blood pressure. The RAAS blockers lower blood pressure through a relaxant effect on the artery, primarily at the level of the endothelium, by interfering with renin and angiotensin, two potent arterial constricting chemicals. Not only is blood pressure lowered, but so is stress on the heart itself. These medications also promote improved blood flow to the kidneys.

The RAAS blockers can be further categorized as either angiotensin converting enzyme (ACE) inhibitors or angiotensin receptor blockers (ARB). All ultimately work by reducing the amount of stimulation to angiotensin receptors, and thereby relax and dilate the arterial wall.

Some of the most common ACE inhibitors are benazepril (Lotensin), captopril (Capoten), enalapril (Vasotec), fosinopril (Monopril), lisinopril (Prinivil, Zestril), quinapril (Accupril), ramipril (Altace) and trandalopril (Mavik). Some of the most common ARB medications are candesartan (Atacand), irbesartan (Avapro), losartan (Cozaar), telmisartan (Micardis) and valsartan (Diovan).

In primary prevention, the ACE inhibitors, and to a lesser extent the ARB medications have proven value in controlling blood pressure. They are valuable in preventing the risk of kidney disease in diabetics. They may be of value in reducing the risk of atherosclerosis through their favorable effects on the endothelium. The HOPE study evaluated the ACE inhibitor ramipril in nearly 10,000 patients with either established CHD or diabetes. Although this was a mixed group of both primary and secondary prevention patients, after five years the risk of MI was reduced by 26 percent, stroke by 32 percent and death by 16 percent. Thus, ACE inhibitors and ARB medications may be of value in primary prevention of CHD.

In the secondary prevention of CHD events, the European Trial on Reduction of Cardiac Events with Perindopril (EUROPA) of 12,000 patients in Europe with established CHD found ACE inhibitor therapy reduced the risk of CHD events recurring, including MI and death by 20 percent. However, the Prevention of Events with Angiotensin Converting Enzyme inhibitor Trial (PEACE) in 8,000 American patients with CHD did not find a benefit. One criticism of the PEACE trial was that it was conducted in lower-risk subjects, and so it is likely they did not derive as much benefit as did the EUROPA trial patients. Thus, the majority of higher risk patients with established CHD should receive ACE inhibitors for secondary prevention.

The data for secondary prevention benefits of ACE inhibitors and ARBs is even more robust in patients who are post-MI and/or have CHF. The Studies of Left Ventricular Dysfunction (SOLVD) and Survival and Ventricular Enlargement (SAVE) trials for ACE inhibitors and the Valsartan in Acute Myocardial Infarction (VALIANT) trial for ARBs showed that these medications significantly reduce the risk of recurrent CHD events and improve life expectancy and heart function in such patients. Thus, either ACE inhibitors or ARBs are essential in the treatment of patients with an EF of less than 40 percent.

The most common side effect of ACE inhibitors is a cough. In most instances, the cough is a nuisance and not a sign of any lung or airway damage or injury. It often improves with continued therapy, but if it does not, switching to an ARB will generally provide the same heart benefit without the cough. In patients with severe sensitivity, both ACE inhibitors and ARBs can precipitate a condition called angioedema, during which the face and neck swell suddenly; it can be fatal if the throat air passages completely close. These medications can also increase blood potassium levels and worsen kidney function.

Antiplatelet Medications. The antiplatelet medications work to inhibit the stickiness of platelets, the primary circulating blood cells that are responsible for clot formation in the artery. Since the ultimate and final trigger for most heart attacks and strokes is the formation of a clump of platelets that form a blood clot in the artery, these medications are extremely effective both in primary prevention as well as secondary prevention of both MI and stroke. There are two types of antiplatelet medications: aspirin and the newer platelet receptor blockers.

1. Aspirin. Aspirin works by blocking platelet clumping. One way platelets trigger clumping together is by generating molecules called thromboxanes internally and then releasing them into the bloodstream. In this state, platelets are called "activated." Thromboxanes trigger activation of even more platelets, resulting in a vicious cycle of more and more platelets clumping together. Aspirin prevents the generation of thromboxanes and so reduces platelet clumping and arterial clots.

Aspirin has been proven to reduce the risk of heart attacks and strokes in secondary prevention. The Second International Study of Infarct Survival (ISIS-2) showed that, following an MI, aspirin reduced the risk of a second MI by 50 percent and reduced the risk of dying by 23 percent. In patients with stable CHD, the Antiplatelet Trialists Collaborative (APTC) showed aspirin reduced the risk of CHD events or death by 25 percent. Aspirin has also been shown to be essential for preventing coronary artery blood clots in patients who have had coronary angioplasty, stents or bypass surgery. Aspirin also improves circulation in patients with PVD, in which atherosclerosis affects the arteries of the legs.

There remains a significant debate about the proper dose of aspirin needed in order to prevent and treat CHD events in patients with known CHD. While it is well established that too low a dose of aspirin increases the risk of CHD events, somewhat paradoxically, so does too high a dose of aspirin. For patients who have had an MI, angioplasty, stents or bypass surgery, the preferred dose of aspirin is between 160 and 325 milligrams per day, which should be continued indefinitely. In most instances,

when other blood thinners are used along with aspirin, the dose
of aspirin is reduced.

For primary prevention, aspirin appears to reduce the risk of
CHD events by about one percent per year. The current AHA
recommendations for aspirin in primary prevention are to
administer 75 milligrams per day if the ten-year Framingham Risk
Score is greater than ten percent and the risk of benefit outweighs
the risk of GI side effects. Based upon the results of the 40,000
women in the Women's Health Study (WHS) and the 22,000 men
in the Physician's Health Study (PHS), the U.S. Preventative
Services Task Force recommendations differ somewhat. They
suggest primary prevention with aspirin in women 55 years of age
or older at a dose of 81 milligrams daily, primarily for stroke prevention. In the WHS, stroke risk was reduced by 17 percent with
aspirin therapy, and there was no change in the risk of MI. In the
PHS, MI risk in men was reduced by 32 percent, and there was
no change in stroke risk. Thus, men over the age of 45 should
take 81 milligrams daily, primarily for MI protection. No mortality benefits to aspirin therapy have been demonstrated in any
large clinical trial for primary prevention.

Keep in mind that even though aspirin is an OTC drug, it is
far from benign. It is a common cause of stomach irritation that
can lead to ulcers and serious GI hemorrhage. Aspirin is acetyl-
salicylic acid, and as an acidic chemical it can be very irritating to
the lining of the stomach. As a blood thinner, aspirin can also
increase the risk of other forms of bleeding. In high doses, aspirin
can also cause kidney damage and a condition called tinnitus, in
which there is a constant ringing in the ears. While true aspirin
allergy is uncommon, when present, it can lead to severe allergic
reactions and even death.

2. Clopidrogel. Clopidrogel (Plavix) is a more potent antiplatelet
medication than aspirin. Unlike aspirin, clopidrogel works to
block the adenosine diphosphate (ADP) receptor on the surface
of platelets. The effect of this is the same as what happens with

aspirin; the platelets are less sticky and less likely to clump together. The platelet-blocking effect of clopidrogel is much more potent and more prolonged than that of aspirin.

Clopidrogel has no established role in primary prevention, but has been extensively studied in secondary prevention. In the Clopidrogel Versus Aspirin in Patients at Risk of Ischemic Events (CAPRIE) study of 20,000 patients with CHD, it was shown to reduce the risk of future CHD events by 10 percent compared to aspirin. The subsequent Clopidrogel in Unstable Angina to Prevent Recurrent Events (CURE) and Clopidrogel as Adjunct Reperfusion Therapy (CLARITY) trials showed the benefits of clopidrogel also extended to patients having an acute coronary syndrome (ACS; either an acute MI or a severe episode of angina). It is effective in preventing clots in patients who have had coronary angioplasty and/or stent procedures. In most patients having had a stent procedure, clopidrogel is used for a minimum of one year. Like aspirin, clopidrogel is effective in stroke prevention and treatment as well as in patients with PVD. Clopidrogel can cause serious bleeding problems, especially from the GI tract.

Alert! Approximately two to fourteen percent of patients are resistant to the antiplatelet effects of clopidrogel because of a genetic variation that alters their metabolism of the drug. There is an ethnic predisposition to this resistance; it is five to ten times more common in blacks and Asians than in Caucasians. Simple blood tests can check for this.

3. Other Antiplatelet Medications. Prasugrel (Effient) and Ticagrelor (Brilinta) are two recently released antiplatelet medications. Both were found in large clinical trials to be superior to clopidrogel in patients treated for ACS. They also work by blocking surface ADP receptors on platelets, but are processed by the body in a manner that makes them more effective and act more rapidly than clopidrogel to block platelet stickiness. In most cases, patients will have had an angioplasty or stent procedure. Prasugrel is not used in patients having had a previous stroke or TIA, since it can increase the risk of brain hemorrhage. Ticagrelor can be used in patients having had an episode of ACS without necessarily having had an angioplasty or stent. Since both are blood thinners, they can substantially increase the risk of bleeding.

Lipid-Modifying Therapy; LDL Lowering

The National Cholesterol Education Program (NCEP) guidelines indicate that the primary target of lipid management in nearly all categories of lipid disorders and CHD risk is the LDL-C level. Medications that lower LDL-C also reduce LDL particle number, Apo B100 content and non-HDL cholesterol levels. Recall from our previous discussions that improvements in these parameters may be even more important in retarding the atherosclerotic process than LDL-C reduction. The NCEP guidelines for the target LDL-C values vary according to the patient's specific risk category and, along with the Apo B100 and non-HDL-C targets, are noted in **table 7.1**.

There is substantial evidence that LDL-C reduction is effective in primary and secondary prevention, as well as in the reversal of atherosclerosis. The evidence is strongest for the use of statin medications as the primary treatment modality by which LDL-C reduction is achieved.

Before discussing the evidence of a benefit in LDL-C reduction and reduced CHD risk, it is worthy to discuss what "normal" LDL-C levels are. The NCEP recommendations of LDL-C targets are based upon two forms of data: (1) epidemiological population data shows reduced CHD risk corresponds to lower LDL-C levels and (2) clinical trials that have shown a linear relationship between LDL-C reduction and CHD risk. The average LDL-C in adults in the United States is 130 mg/dL. Since CHD is present in almost half of all adults by the time they reach age 50, the average level of LDL-C is clearly not a protective level. Of note, an LDL-C of 130 mg/dL is indeed the NCEP-recommended target LDL-C level for patients at low and moderate CHD risk.

There is in fact considerable evidence that suggests that optimal physiological levels of LDL-C are different from our current targets. Anthropological data indicates that when our ancestors lived in hunter-gatherer societies, the incidence of CHD was extremely low. While other illnesses caused a reduced life expectancy in these populations, many individuals still lived well into their seventh and eighth decades. Analysis of fossilized tissue samples from some of these societies has revealed that LDL-C levels were, on average, 50–75 mg/dL. The LDL-C levels in healthy babies born today are 30–70 mg/dL. Healthy, wild adult primates have LDL-C levels of 40–80 mg/dL. In fact, modern humans are the only adult mammals, excluding some domesticated animals that have a mean LDL-C level over 80 mg/dL. Thus, there may be discordance between what is genetically determined to be optimal lipid levels and what we have currently achieved.

Clinical studies convincingly demonstrate that halting plaque progression and plaque regression occurs only when LDL-C levels are reduced to 80 mg/dL or below. It is also at these levels that other beneficial effects in the artery occur, including reduced inflammation, thrombosis and oxidation. Furthermore, at low LDL levels, the adverse impact and significance of an elevated Lp(a) level disappears.

> **Illumination:** Since cholesterol is vital to many biological processes, the question of how low is too low arises? While it is true that malnourished individuals and cancer patients develop low LDL-C levels that are associated with poor health outcomes, naturally occurring low LDL-C levels are indeed associated with reduced CHD risk and improved longevity. If our body is originally programmed to function at an optimal LDL-C level of 50–70 mg/dL, perhaps this is the range that should be considered ideal.

Based upon these findings, many atherosclerosis experts believe patients are not better served by trying to achieve any specific LDL-C threshold as a target based upon an assessment of their CHD risk category. Instead, for both primary and secondary prevention in all individuals, LDL-C should be reduced by 30 percent and 50 percent respectively, and for reversal, LDL-C should be brought to less than 80 mg/dL.

Statins. These are the most widely prescribed medications in the world. Currently, nearly 40 million people in the United States are on statins. Their use is increasing, and 25 percent more people take statins now than in 2007. Before it became generic in 2012, Atorvastatin, marketed as Lipitor was the best-selling drug in the world, with annual sales of nearly 13 billion dollars.

Statins work by blocking the manufacture of cholesterol, which is controlled by the liver enzyme HMG-CoA reductase. When this enzyme is blocked, not only is less cholesterol made, the liver is stimulated to make more LDL surface receptors, which help remove the LDL lipid particles from the bloodstream.

Statins are the most effective way to lower LDL-C and have been extensively studied in both primary and secondary prevention, as well as in reversal of CHD. The LDL-C lowering effect varies according to the potency of the statin but typically begins within two weeks of the start of treatment. The most effective statins will lower LDL-C by up to 60 percent at maximum doses, and the least potent statins will lower LDL-C by 25 percent at the lowest doses. Statins also lower Apo B100 and LDL particle numbers, although not to the same degree as they lower LDL-C. In addition to their LDL-C lowering effects, they also modestly lower triglycerides by 15–30 percent and raise HDL-C by three to ten percent. Statins have no effect on Lp(a).

Statins also have what are called pleiotropic effects, meaning beneficial actions above and beyond their lipid effects. These include reducing arterial inflammation, as shown by a reduction in CRP levels. They may improve endothelial function, reduce lipid oxidation and stabilize vulnerable plaque. By virtue of these non-lipid effects, there is some evidence that statin therapy may be beneficial in a variety of non-CHD patients, such as those with CHF, artificial heart valves, arthritis, infection, and sepsis. There are studies that indicate that all statins may not be alike with respect to their pleiotropic benefits.

Statins have been associated with a number of adverse effects. There does not appear to be any one statin that is more or less likely to cause side effects than another, although there does appear to be some relation between dose and occurrence for certain side effects. The most common is the occurrence of muscle aches, a condition known as myalgia, reported by two to five percent of patients taking statins. In rare cases (five in 100,000), muscle aches can progress to muscle damage through inflammation, or myositis. In severe and even rarer (less than one in 500,000) instances, statin-induced myositis can lead to permanent kidney damage and even death (one in ten million). In many cases, myalgia can be managed by switching to a different statin, reducing the dose and even using CoQ10 supplementation. Certain predisposing factors to the development of statin-induced muscle problems have been identified (**table 13.1**). If these apply to you, your risk of having muscle problems is higher.

Table 13.1
Conditions that Increase the Risk
of Muscle Problems with Statin Therapy

Increasing Age
Female Sex
Chronic Kidney Disease
Chronic Liver Abnormalities
Hypothyroidism
Consumption of Grapefruit or Pomegranate Juice
Consumption of Alcohol
Use of Multiple Medications; especially Gemfibrozil
High Intensity Exercise

Statins can increase blood sugar and even hasten the development of diabetes. They can cause minor abnormalities in liver function, although as of yet there are no documented cases of liver failure. On the other hand, statins have actually been shown to improve kidney function by five to ten percent. They can cause abdominal pain, constipation, gas or cramps. They have been associated with alterations in memory and cognitive function.

Other medications that are metabolized by the liver may affect and also be affected by certain statins. Grapefruit juice affects the metabolism of statins, since it contains a chemical that affects certain digestive enzymes. Since this effect can be prolonged, grapefruit juice should be avoided by those taking statins.

The first available statin was Lovastatin (Mevacor), released in 1987. In addition to this drug, there are six other currently available statins in the United States; atorvastatin (Lipitor), fluvastatin (Lescol), pitivastatin (Livalo), pravastatin (Pravachol), rosuvastatin (Crestor) and simvastatin (Zocor). Cervistatin (Baycol) was pulled from the market in 2001 because of an unexpectedly high rate of muscle injury and kidney failure.

The statin medications can be classified in various ways that help determine how they are used. The most common classification systems take into account (1) whether they are naturally derived from fungi or synthetically made, (2) half-life and duration of effect, (3) whether they are metabolized by the liver or not, (4) water or fat solubility, (5) generic or brand and (6) potency. Some of these distinguishing characteristics are presented in **table 13.2**.

Table 13.2
Important Characteristics that
Distinguish Individual Statins

Statin	Dose range	Range of LDL Lowering	Liver Metabolism	Natural (Fungal) or Synthetic
Lovastatin	20-80 mg	20-40%	Yes	Natural
Simvastatin	10-80*mg	25-45%	Yes	Natural
Pravastatin	20-80 mg	25-45%	No	Natural
Fluvastatin	40-80 mg	25-35%	Yes	Synthetic
Atorvastatin	10-80 mg	35-50%	Yes	Synthetic
Rosuvastatin	5-40 mg	35-55%	No	Synthetic
Pitivastatin	2-4 mg	40-50%	No	Synthetic

*= the 80 mg dose of Simvastatin is no longer recommended

Based upon these characteristics, certain stains are preferred in certain situations. For instance, pravastatin and fluvastatin are the preferred statin for kidney patients. Atorvastatin and rosuvastatin are the preferred statins for the greatest LDL-C lowering potency. Pravastatin and pitivastatin have very few medication interactions, and so are preferred for patients on complex or extensive medication regimens. Lovastatin and simvastatin are among the oldest statins and, by virtue of no ongoing patent, are also the least expensive.

For primary prevention data, the four largest statin trials were the Air Force/Texas Coronary Atherosclerosis Prevention Studies (AFCAPS/

TexCAPS) using lovastatin, the West of Scotland Coronary Prevention Study (WOSCOPS) using pravastatin, the Anglo-Scandanavian Cardiac Outcomes Trial (ASCOT) using atorvastatin, and the Justification for the use of Statins in Prevention: an Intervention Trail Evaluating Rosuvastatin (JUPITER). These trials all studied thousands of individuals with elevated LDL-C levels and no known CHD for several years. Statin treatment groups were compared to individuals receiving optimal diet therapy. The studies all showed very comparable results: on average a 30–40 percent risk reduction in CHD events. However, none showed a reduction in mortality rates. The number needed to treat (NNT), which is viewed as a benchmark of the efficacy of a medication, represents the number of individuals who would need to be treated for one single patient to derive a benefit. In almost all of the primary prevention trials, the five-year NNT was about 50.

> **Illumination:** Comparing other CHD prevention methods to statin therapy by NNT is instructive. For primary prevention, the average NNT for statins is 50 patients. Other primary prevention strategies for CHD perform much worse; treatment of hypertension has a five-year NNT of 90–140, and aspirin prophylaxis has a five-year NNT of 346 for men and 426 for women.

The JUPITER trial attempted to further refine risk assessment in primary prevention by requiring individuals to have abnormal lipids and an elevated CRP level to be included in the study. In this study, the risk reductions were more robust, averaging 40–50 percent for most types of CHD events. For this reason, the study was actually stopped two years earlier than planned, as it was considered unethical to continue to offer at-risk patients placebo therapy when the treatment group was deriving such significant benefits. Despite the robust drop in CHD event rates, there was still no mortality benefit. The overall five-year NNT was reduced to 20. However, two subgroups, patients with Framingham Risk Scores in excess of 10 percent and those with a family history of premature CHD, derived even greater benefit had five-year NNT values of 14 and nine, respectively.

The Collaborative Atorvastatin Diabetes Study (CARDS) evaluated primary prevention of CHD in 2,000 diabetics without known CHD, ages 40–72 years, in the U.K. Although it was called a primary prevention trial, the study group had diabetes, which is considered a CHD risk equivalent, and so the participants likely were a higher risk group than true primary prevention patients. Subjects were randomized to receive either a placebo or atorvastatin over a four-year period. The outcomes in the atorvastatin group were impressive, showing a 36 percent reduction in CHD events, a 31 percent reduction in need for PCI or CABG procedures and a 45 percent reduction in strokes. This is the only statin "primary prevention" trial to show a mortality benefit, with a 27 percent reduction in mortality in the group receiving atorvastatin compared to a placebo.

For secondary prevention, the largest statin trials are the Cholesterol and Recurrent Trial (CARE) and Long-term Intervention with Pravastatin in Ischemic Disease Trial (LIPID) using pravastatin, the Scandinavian Simvastatin Survival Study (4S) and Heart Protection Study (HPS) using simvastatin and the Treatment to New Targets (TNT) and Incremental Decrease in Endpoints through Aggressive Lipid Lowering (IDEAL) statin-comparison trials. These trials were also conducted in thousands of patients over several years. They showed an average of 30–40 percent risk reductions, more robust results than the primary prevention trials, since they were conducted in patients who had established CHD and thus were at higher risk of having CHD events. Most of these trials also showed reduced mortality rates due to heart disease in the group taking statin medications. The five-year NNT values in these studies were in the range of 12–30 patients.

One large statin trial has specifically looked at the question of whether statins reduce the risk of stroke or TIA. The Stroke Prevention by Aggressive Reduction in Cholesterol Levels (SPARCL) trial evaluated atorvastatin compared to placebo in 5,000 patients with a history of stroke or TIA within the previous one to six months, who did not have known coronary artery disease. After five years of follow-up, LDL-C levels dropped to 70 mg/dL in treated patients, the risk of stroke was reduced by 16 percent, the risk of all CHD events was reduced by 20 percent, and there was no change in mortality rates. The patients who achieved the lowest

LDL-C levels, typically at or below 70 mg/dL, derived the most benefit, an almost 30 percent reduction in rate of recurrent stroke.

Illumination: Physician, heal thyself; Luke 4:23. Cardiologists are sold on the benefits of statins. Recent surveys show that 90 percent of cardiologists take statins themselves, often at lower LDL-C levels than for which they would prescribe for their patients. Having access to free samples certainly eliminates one hurdle.

However, setting a good example for their patients is not something that doctors and nurses do particularly well. The Physicians Health Study found 38 percent of male physicians had a BMI over 25 kg/m^2 and six percent had a BMI over 30 kg/m^2. The Nurses' Health Study found 23 percent of women nurses had a BMI over 25 kg/m^2 and five percent had a BMI over 32 kg/m^2. In a Swiss survey, only 57 percent of physicians said they exercised regularly. Multiple studies indicate that patients are two to three times more likely to accept and follow counseling on lifestyle management if their physicians are normal weight.

A number of studies with statins have shown that these medications can prevent the progression of plaque and in some instances cause plaque regression. These studies have used a variety of imaging tests, including coronary angiography, carotid intimal medial thickness (cIMT) and intracoronary ultrasound (ICUS). Although highly invasive and complex to perform, the last technique appears to be the most sensitive, specific, and has the most rigorous standard for evaluating changes in coronary plaque. In the Reversal of Atherosclerosis with Aggressive Lipid Lowering (REVERSAL) trial of 500 patients studied by ICUS, when LDL-C levels of 80 mg/dL were achieved with atorvastatin, plaque progression was halted. In the 'A Study to Evaluate the Effects of Rosuvastatin on Intravascular Ultrasound-Derived Coronary Artery Atheroma Burden (ASTEROID)' trial of 350 patients, lowering of LDL-C to 60 mg/dL, along with a modest rise in HDL-C by 15 percent, was associated with plaque reversal in 75 percent of patients by an average of six to eight percent of the original plaque burden.

Bile Acid Sequestrants. Bile acid sequestrants (BAS) are also known as bile acid resins. They reduce LDL-C by binding the cholesterol-rich bile salts that enter the intestine when secreted by the gall bladder to aid in digestion. When these bile acids are bound by the BAS, cholesterol is excreted in the stool and not allowed to reenter the circulation. The most commonly used BAS medications are cholestyramine (Questran), colesevelam (Welchol) and colestipol (Colestid). They can be taken as powders mixed in water or juice, or as tablets.

These medications are much less potent than statins and will typically lower LDL-C by 10–20 percent. They have no effect on HDL-C and may actually increase triglycerides. When combined with statins, they provide an additional 15 percent reduction in LDL-C than with statin therapy alone. Their clinical efficacy was demonstrated in several trials, including the Lipid Research Clinics-Coronary Primary Prevention Trial (LRC-CPPT) and Familial Atherosclerosis Treatment Study (FATS).

Their main side effects occur in the GI tract and include constipation, bloating, nausea, pain and gas. In fact, less than half of all patients prescribed these medications can stick with them because of the prominent GI side effects. GI side effects appear to be less pronounced with the newest agent, colesevelam. BAS medications can also interfere with absorption of other medications, so most medications need to be taken at least one hour apart from the BAS dose. They reduce the absorption of fat-soluble vitamins, so these usually need to be supplemented. They can also cause liver damage.

Ezetemibe. Ezetemibe (Zetia) is also an LDL-C lowering medication. It works by blocking a transport protein, the Niemann-Pick C1-like protein, found in intestinal cells. This protein is necessary for the absorption of cholesterol. By itself, it is a relatively weak drug, typically reducing LDL-C by only 15 percent. However, when combined with a statin, ezetemibe can provide an additional 20 percent effectiveness in lowering LDL-C over and above statin therapy alone. Thus, when ezetemibe is combined with the most effective statin, LDL-C may drop by 80 percent. It is available in combination therapy with simvastatin as the brand medication Vytorin. Ezetemibe has almost no effect on triglycerides or HDL-C.

Ezetemibe is very well tolerated, although there are rare reports of liver and muscle problems. When combined with statin therapy, the risk of liver abnormalities is increased up to three-fold, compared to statin therapy alone. No clinical trials using ezetemibe alone for primary or secondary prevention have been done. The Ezetemibe and Simvastatin in Hypercholesterolemia Enhances Atherosclerosis Regression (ENHANCE) trial using ezetemibe combined with simvastatin to assess plaque reversal found no benefit in retarding or reducing plaque growth with ezetemibe.

Lipid-Modifying Therapy: Treatment of Mixed Dyslipidemia

These medications have affects on multiple lipid particles. They are especially important, as two-thirds of all people with lipid disorders have the condition of mixed dyslipidemia. In this condition, the lipid disorder is some combination of high LDL-C, high triglycerides and low HDL-C. In most instances, the medications used to counteract mixed dyslipidemia are not selected purely for their LDL-C lowering affects, even though some have significant ability to lower LDL-C. Instead, the goal in using these drugs is either to lower triglycerides or to raise HDL-C, or they are used as second-line drugs for lowering LDL-C because the patient cannot tolerate other LDL-C lowering medications, or as combination therapy to achieve further lowering of LDL-C.

The effect of high triglycerides on CHD risk remains controversial. Thus, lowering triglycerides to reduce CHD risk is of unproven benefit. However, elevated triglycerides appear to be a marker of an atherogenic state. More of the atherogenic Apo B100-containing particles are present when triglycerides are high. Also, less of the anti-atherogenic HDL particles are present. High triglyceride levels are a marker for both metabolic syndrome and diabetes, both of which increase CHD risk. High triglyceride levels are also often associated with a high number of LDL particles, since there are more small, dense LDL particles, even though LDL-C levels may be normal. In general, the higher triglyceride levels are at the start of treatment, the greater the benefits with triglyceride-reducing therapies.

Many HDL-C population studies indicate that HDL-C levels correlate negatively with CHD risk: as HDL-C levels rise, CHD risk drops. Some plaque reversal studies have found a strong association between rising HDL-C and regression of plaque. Data from clinical trials remains inconclusive about whether interventions that raise HDL-C can reduce CHD risk or mortality.

Fish Oil. For the same reasons that fish oil supplements and consumption of omega-3 fatty acids from fatty fish are an important component of many heart-healthy diet plans, prescription fish oil supplements are very commonly used to assist in the management of CHD risk and lipid treatment. There is strong evidence that prescription fish oil preparations are of benefit in both preventing and treating CHD. Until recently, the only approved prescription formulation of fish oil in the United States was Lovaza, a combination of EPA and DHA omega-3 fatty acids in a total dose of 850 milligrams per capsule. In July 2012, Vascepa, an ultra-pure formulation of primarily EPA was also approved. Both Lovaza and Vascepa are indicated and approved by the FDA for treatment of very high triglycerides.

Prescription fish oil has been shown to reduce triglycerides and Lp(a) and to increase HDL-C. In patients with high triglyceride levels, the maximum dose of four grams per day will reduce VLDL and triglycerides on average by 45 percent. The combination omega-3 fatty acids in Lovaza may increase LDL-C, especially in patients who have very high triglycerides. The mechanism by which fish oil exerts its lipid benefits is likely through reduced liver production of triglycerides.

One of the largest trials to demonstrate a benefit of prescription fish oil was the GISSI-P study, which looked at more than 11,324 men and women in Italy who had known CHD. Participants who consumed just one fish oil capsule per day reduced their risk of MI and sudden death by 30 percent over one year. This was likely a result of fish oil's effect on stabilizing the electrical system of the heart.

The Japanese EPA lipid intervention trial evaluated the use of prescription fish oil containing only EPA at a dose of 1,800 milligrams per day, along with a low dose of statin therapy, in over 18,000 patients with established CHD who had been followed for five years. There was a 19 percent reduction in risk of a future CHD event in those who took combination therapy, compared to those who took just statin therapy. One unique property of EPA alone is that it does not cause a rise in LDL-C, as can sometimes occur with the currently available EPA and DHA combinations. This property may offer a potential advantage of Vascepa over Lovaza. In preliminary studies, Vascepa also reduced LDL particle number, Apo B100, small, dense LDL particles and CRP levels.

In 2007, another Japanese study in which EPA was administered to men without CHD, but who had high blood sugar levels, found less plaque and intimal thickening as well as improved blood flow in the carotid arteries compared to those not receiving EPA. Two review articles in 2006 evaluated all published studies of fish oil. Both concluded that scientific evidence supported that regular fish oil consumption was associated with reduced mortality and CHD events. Thus, prescription fish oil has proven benefits in improving blood lipids, particularly in subjects with high triglycerides or low HDL-C. Fish oil is also effective in the secondary prevention of CHD events and in the primary prevention of atherosclerosis.

Side effects related to fish oil are primarily GI in nature. It can cause a fishy odor to the breath, indigestion and diarrhea. Another potential problem is that by virtue of its blood thinning properties, fish oil may increase the risk of bleeding. This is more of a theoretical concern than a practical one, and typically becomes an issue only if patients take other blood thinners or are undergoing major surgery.

Niacin. Niacin affects all lipoproteins, but is one of the best currently available ways to raise HDL-C. Niacin blocks the breakdown of fats in adipose tissue, and so decreases free fatty acids in the bloodstream. This decrease in free fatty acids causes the liver to make less VLDL, LDL and cholesterol, and so all of these lipids are lowered. The lowering of VLDL has a reciprocal effect on HDL particles, which are caused to increase. Niacin may also retard removal of the main apolipoprotein in the HDL particle, Apo A1, thus making more Apo A1 available for HDL synthesis.

Prescription niacin is available as immediate-release niacin and the more commonly prescribed extended-release niacin, marketed as Niaspan. Both forms are better absorbed with food. Niacin can cause liver abnormalities, aggravate gout by increasing uric acid and cause GI problems and ulcers. Niacin may increase blood sugar in diabetics.

As for OTC niacin preparations, the main side effect of prescription extended and immediate release niacin is flushing and itching of the skin. This is caused by the release of a family of chemicals called prostaglandins. These cause the capillaries under the skin to dilate, making the skin tingle, sting, and turn red. It is considered a nuisance side effect rather than a sign of any toxicity of the chemical. With continued use, the itching and flushing resolve. Taking aspirin 30 minutes before taking the niacin will significantly reduce the symptoms, as will taking the niacin with a low-fat snack, avoiding alcohol and taking the niacin before going to bed at night. Immediate release niacin causes more flushing than the extended-release form of Niaspan.

Typically, therapeutic doses of niacin will lower triglycerides by 20–40 percent and LDL-C by 10–20 percent and raise HDL-C by 15–30 percent. Whereas the triglyceride and LDL-C lowering effects occur within a few days, the HDL-C raising effects can take several months. Other lipid benefits include lowering of Lp(a), small, dense LDL, Apo B, and the LDL particle number. Niacin also increases the proportion of the most beneficial type of HDL, the large HDL-2 subtypes. When combined with statin therapy, the favorable lipid effects of niacin are even more pronounced. However, the risk of toxicity, especially muscle and kidney damage, is also increased.

Scientific data studied over a 30-year period has shown multiple benefits from niacin intake. There is substantial evidence that immediate-release niacin reduces the risk of CHD. It has been shown to prevent a first heart attack, prevent a recurrent heart attack in patients who have already had CHD and to reverse atherosclerosis. In the Coronary Drug Project (CDP), completed in 1975, niacin treatment for six years in over 8,000 men after a first MI reduced the risk of recurrent MI, death, and stoke by 27 percent. A 25-year follow-up study of the same patients in the CDP trial that was recently published found a 14 percent reduced mortality rate in the niacin patients. Other studies have also established niacin's value in reducing all CHD events.

Multiple imaging studies have shown niacin may promote regression of atherosclerosis. Most recently, in 2009, the Arterial Biology for the Investigation of the Treatment Effects of Reducing Cholesterol 6: HDL and LDL Treatment Strategies in Atherosclerosis (ARBITER 6 HALTS) trial demonstrated that extended-release niacin added to statin therapy reduced carotid intimal thickness more effectively than the LDL-C lowering drug ezetemibe when added to statin therapy. A recent meta-analysis of 11 randomized clinical trials of immediate- and extended-release niacin confirmed that niacin reduces the risk of CHD events and the progression of atherosclerosis in nearly all types of patients studied.

The Atherothrombosis Intervention in Metabolic Syndrome with Low HDL/High Triglycerides: Impact on Global Health Outcomes (AIM-HIGH) trial published in 2011 has called into question the beneficial effects of extended-release niacin for all patient types. In this study of over 3,000 patients for 36 months, those with well-controlled LDL-C levels on statin therapy and known CHD derived no additional benefit from niacin, despite increasing their HDL-C levels. For unexplained reasons, in numbers not statistically significant, twice as many patients receiving niacin had strokes.

Fibrates. Fibrates are among the best drugs for reducing triglycerides. They typically will reduce triglycerides by 20–50 percent. They also raise HDL-C, usually by 10–15 percent. However, by themselves they have only a slight effect on LDL-C, an average lowering of 10–15 percent. They decrease the proportion of small, dense LDL particles and may lower Lp(a) slightly. They affect lipids by activating a group of receptors on the liver called PPAR-alpha receptors. This increases removal of triglycerides by activating the enzyme that is primarily responsible for triglyceride degradation, lipoprotein lipase.

The most commonly used fibrates are fenofibrate (Tricor, Trilipix, Antara, Lofibra and Triglide) and gemfibrozil (Lopid). Fibrates can potentiate the effects of blood thinners like warfarin (Coumadin). They can cause GI problems as well as increase the risk of gallstones. When combined with statins, as they often are, they increase the risk of liver and muscle abnormalities; this is much more common with gemfibrozil than the fenofibrate derivatives.

The clinical trials of fibrates in reducing CHD risk have yielded mixed results. The Helsinki Heart Study (HHS) found that gemfibrozil reduced CHD events through a rise in HDL-C independent of a lowering of LDL-C. However, most of the benefit was confined to patients with elevated triglycerides or who were obese. The Veterans Administration-High Density Lipoprotein Intervention Trial (VA-HIT) also evaluated gemfibrozil and found raising HDL-C was associated with reduced CHD events and death. However, the rise in HDL-C accounted for only about one-quarter of the benefit.

The Bezafibrate Infarction Prevention (BIP) trial, conducted in Israel, used bezafibrate (not available in the United States). It found the drug conferred no overall benefit on CHD risk, despite an 18 percent rise in HDL-C. However, patients with metabolic syndrome and high triglycerides did seem to derive a modest reduction of CHD risk. The 10,000-subject Fenofibrate Intervention and Event Lowering in Diabetes (FIELD) trial of diabetics using fenofibrate found only a two percent rise in HDL-C and no clinical benefit. However, there was a 30 percent reduction in diabetes-related retinal problems. There was a design flaw in the trial in that twice as many patients in the placebo group compared to the fibrate group were started on statin therapy during the study. This may have confounded the results of this study.

The Action to Control Cardiovascular Risk in Diabetes (ACCORD) trial of over 5,000 patients with diabetes found no overall benefit from the addition of fibrate therapy to baseline statin therapy on CHD risk or mortality over five years. However, the group with the highest triglyceride and lowest HDL-C levels derived significant benefit, showing a 30 percent CHD risk reduction. As was observed in the FIELD trial, subjects receiving fibrates had a drop in diabetes-related retinal problems, in this case of 40 percent.

Thus, the CHD benefits remain a matter of significant debate. A recent meta-analysis of multiple pooled trials in over 45,000 patients found a ten percent risk reduction in CHD events and no mortality benefit. The same study also showed fibrate therapy reduced patients' risk of needing future heart procedures such as bypass surgery or angioplasty. Fibrate therapy also reduced the risk of kidney problems and progressive atherosclerosis changes in the retina of the eye.

Lipid-Modifying Therapy: Advanced and Novel Treatments

New medications for the treatment of lipid abnormalities remain a priority for pharmaceutical companies and health care professionals. The existing therapies continue to have problems with limited effectiveness and side effects. Given the burden of CHD, the potential economic incentives for drug companies and clinical incentives for patients and health care providers are enormous.

LDL Apheresis. In the technique of LDL apheresis, the patient's blood is cleansed of LDL particles by passing through a cleansing apparatus similar to a dialysis machine. It is generally reserved for patients with homozygous familial hypercholesterolemia and some patients with the less severe heterozygous variety who either do not respond to medications to lower LDL-C or in whom medications are contraindicated. It is a safe procedure that can reduce LDL-C by 60–80 percent. However, it is expensive and inconvenient, as it requires two hours per session and must be repeated every one to two weeks.

Squalene Synthase Inhibitors. Like statins, these medications work in the cholesterol production chain. However, they work downstream and do not lower levels of CoQ10. Thus, they may be attractive, as they offer the hope of being as effective as statins, while having fewer muscle side effects. Early clinical trials indicated some increased risk of liver problems. However, one drug, lapaquistat, is now in clinical trials.

ACAT inhibitors. The enzyme acyl-CoA cholesterol acyl transferase (ACAT) plays a role in regulating cholesterol absorption and manufacture. Laboratory studies indicate that blocking the ACAT enzyme has been shown to lower cholesterol levels and also reduce the level of plaque. Two drugs that reached clinical trials were pactimibe and avasimibe, but they were not found to be effective and in fact appeared to increase plaque burden. This area remains an area of active research interest.

MTP Inhibitors. Microsomal transport protein (MTP) is necessary for the liver to make VLDL particles. In people with the genetic defect abetalipoproteinemia, in which this enzyme is lacking, the levels of Apo B100 are extremely low, and CHD is extremely uncommon. Early trials indicate that medications that block the MTP enzyme reduce LDL-C by 50 percent. There are two drugs in this category that have reached human trials, lomitapide and implitapide. However, the findings of an increase in liver problems and poor tolerability have limited development of these compounds.

Apo B Antisense. In this therapy, chemicals that interfere with the synthesis of RNA, which mediates the generation of the Apo B100 protein, are administered to reduce Apo B100 levels. In a recent clinical trial, administration of such a compound once a week by subcutaneous injection reduced LDL-C in patients with familial hypercholesterolemia by 50 percent. Apo B100 levels and Lp(a) levels dropped by 25 percent. The drug in this category that has been investigated the most is mipomersen. It remains in clinical development but has been associated with liver problems.

PCSK9 Inhibitors. The gene PCSK9 is known to be defective in a number of populations. Especially in African Americans, a defect of this gene is believed to be protective against the development of CHD. On the other hand, increased activity of this gene has been shown to reduce the LDL-C lowering effect of statins. Inhibitors of the PCSK9 gene offer a new approach of targeted gene therapy in the management of lipid disorders.

Niacin with Laropripant. A new product, laropripant, has been developed that is an inhibitor of prostaglandin receptors. It has been shown to reduce the intensity of niacin-induced flushing. Early studies indicate that it is well tolerated, and it is currently being studied in a large trial of niacin use in patients with low HDL-C levels, called the Heart Protection Study2—Treatment of HDL to Reduce the Incidence of Vascular Events (HPS2-THRIVE), results from which are expected in 2014. Since flushing is responsible for most of the intolerance associated with niacin, and niacin offers the potential for safely raising HDL-C with some already well-established clinical outcomes, this product may be of value.

HDL Infusions. The most direct benefit of raising HDL levels in clinical trials has been provided by studies in which subjects with known CHD were given infusions of HDL. In one study, 57 subjects received infusions of a type of HDL containing the genetic variation of the HDL apolipoprotein A1$_{Milano}$. This particular type of Apo A1 mutation has been discovered in a cluster of individuals in northern Italy, who have been found to have virtually no CHD. Serum taken from these individuals containing the purified Apo A1$_{Milano}$ HDL was infused at weekly intervals. Remarkably, after just five weeks, subjects with severe coronary plaque showed signs of significant plaque regression assessed by intravascular ultrasound.

CETP Inhibitors. The exchange of cholesterol between HDL, VLDL and LDL in the bloodstream is a continuous and ever-present process that is mediated by the enzyme cholesterol ester transfer protein (CETP). When CETP is blocked, HDL-C levels rise significantly, by up to 100 percent. This finding has fueled an aggressive search for compounds that can do this safely and effectively.

The first compound studied in a large clinical trial was torcetrapib. The Investigation of Lipid Level Management to understand its Impact in Atherosclerosis Events (ILLUMINATE) trial included 15,000 patients who had CHD or diabetes. The trial was stopped in 2006 after only 18 months of follow-up because subjects receiving torcetrapib had a one and one-half times higher rate of death than control subjects. These patients also had higher blood pressures. Although the results of this trial tempered the enthusiasm for CETP inhibition, a subset of patients in this trial that showed the greatest increases in HDL-C levels were found to have significant regression in the level of plaque.

Thus, newer and, one hopes, safer agents for CETP inhibition are currently being investigated. Two new agents, dalcetrapib and anacetrapib are currently in clinical trials and show promise as being effective agents to raise HDL-C without the toxic effects that were observed with torcetrapib. Early data indicates that dalcetrapib increases HDL-C by 35 percent and reduces LDL-C by 10 percent. However, after preliminary results showed no clinical benefit, a large clinical trial evaluating dalcetrapib was stopped early in May, 2012 by the trial sponsor. Anacetrapib has been shown to raise HDL-C by 140 percent, and reduce LDL-C by 40 percent. A large trial to determine its clinical benefit is still ongoing. Neither compound has yet shown evidence of blood pressure rise or other toxic effects of the type that occurred with torcetrapib.

Chapter 14

Special Populations:

Unless You Are a Middle-Aged White Guy,
This Means You ...

THE HARMFUL CONSEQUENCES and life-changing effects of CHD (coronary heart disease) span across race, sex, age and socioeconomic class divisions. However, there are many aspects of CHD that are affected and distinguished by the sex, race and age of the individual. In this chapter, we will discuss some of the unique concerns of CHD prevention, diagnosis and treatment in women and in different age and ethnic groups. We will also discuss the approach to secondary prevention in the most critically ill type of CHD patient: the individual who has already suffered and survived a potentially fatal acute cardiac event and has what is called acute coronary syndrome (ACS).

Women

While death rates for men over the last 30 years due to CHD in the United States have declined by 20 percent, there has been no like decline in death rates for women. In fact, for at least the last 20 years, the number of women dying from CHD has exceeded men. Women are twice as likely as men to die during the first few weeks after a heart attack. It is only in the last five years that we have seen a drop in mortality rates in women from

CHD. What are the reasons for the disparity in the incidence and severity of CHD in women?

> **Alert!** Contrary to popular perception, the leading cause of death in women is not cancer but CHD. One out of 25 women will develop breast cancer; one in 12 women will die of breast cancer; one in two women fears dying of breast cancer. Compare these statistics to those for CHD: one in three women will develop CHD; one in two women will die due to CHD; only one in 25 women fears dying of CHD. CHD in women causes more deaths than the next seven causes of death combined.

Awareness. A significant barrier to the identification and treatment of CHD in women is lack of awareness. One common misconception is that only older women develop CHD. While it is true that women develop heart problems later in life than men, by the time a woman reaches the age of 45 her risk of CHD is nearly equal to that of a man. From that point on, as many, if not more women as men develop CHD. The rate of CHD in women doubles after menopause.

The problem of lack of awareness affects not only patients but also the medical community. In one recent survey of female patients, 70 percent of women stated that their physician had never discussed CHD or risk factors for CHD with them, even though it is well known that women are more likely to have multiple CHD risk factors than men.

As a result of public perception and lack of awareness in the medical community, women are more frequently underdiagnosed with CHD. Women have more atypical symptoms of CHD. This means that instead of the classic "elephant sitting on the chest" type of chest pain that accompanies an MI or episode of angina in men, women more frequently experience symptoms such as back and neck pain, shortness of breath, nausea, vomiting, indigestion and fatigue when they develop angina or an MI. Women more frequently have silent MIs. Two out of three women who die of an MI have no symptoms. Women more frequently have abnormal ECGs and more often have false readings on stress tests. As we will later show, these issues directly relate to the lower rate of effective treatments that are administered to women and the poorer outcomes of CHD-related illnesses in women.

Female CHD Risk factors. The NCEP guidelines for lipid management do not differentiate women and men. LDL-C targets are the same and are based on estimates of CHD risk or evidence of current CHD diagnoses. However, certain risk calculators appear to be more specific to, and accurate in, women, such as the previously discussed Reynolds Risk Score. Also, other lipid parameters beyond LDL-C appear to be more important in women than men.

In women, both the Framingham trial and the Lipid Research Clinics trial have shown that HDL-C and triglyceride levels appear to have a greater impact on CHD risk than men. For women, CHD risk and mortality are three to four times higher if HDL-C level is under 50 mg/dL, compared to HDL-C levels above 50 mg/dL. For triglycerides, every 100-mg/dL rise increases CHD risk three times more in women than it does in men. An elevated Lp(a), the "heart attack protein" that is attached to the LDL particle, is of greater significance in women than it is in men. In the HERS study, Lp(a) was noted to be an independent predictor of CHD risk in post-menopausal women but was not for age-matched men.

Women and men differ in lipoprotein levels in two major ways. The first is that early in life, women tend to have HDL-C levels that are, on average, 10 mg/dL higher than their age-matched male counterparts. Pre-menopausal women also have a higher proportion of the large, buoyant HDL-2, the most protective type of HDL, than do men. The second difference is that women's lipid levels change significantly around the time of menopause. This is believed to be the reason behind a sharp increased in CHD risk and poorer CHD outcomes in post-menopausal women.

At the time of menopause, total cholesterol, LDL-C and triglyceride levels all precipitously spike to values that are on average ten percent higher than they were pre-menopause. There are also adverse changes in Apo B100 levels, LDL particle number and LDL particle size after menopause. The HDL-C in women starts to gradually decline about 20 months before menopause, and continues to do so post-menopause, so that it is typically

20 percent lower one year after menopause compared to what it was two years before menopause. The type of HDL particle also changes after menopause from the more protective large, buoyant HDL-2 to the less protective, smaller type of HDL-3. These lipid changes are caused by a reduction in estrogen levels and their effects on the lipid-generating machinery in the liver.

Other changes in atherosclerosis risk also occur around the time of menopause. These include increased endothelial dysfunction and inflammation. CRP levels usually rise after menopause. Data from the Women's Health Study (WHS) indicates that CRP as a marker of inflammation carries much more significance in women than it does in men.

Obesity is a more prominent risk factor in women than in men. This is partly because women tend to have the most atherogenic type of obesity, central obesity, much more often than men. Obesity in women is also more likely to be associated with metabolic syndrome, which is itself associated with both an increased risk and severity of CHD. Also, diabetes is more common in women, which is a major CHD risk factor. Of special concern is the fact that black and Hispanic women have the highest and also the fastest rising incidence of obesity, metabolic syndrome and diabetes of any sex or ethnic group. Other risk factors like stress, anxiety and depression affect women differently than men and with increased frequency and severity.

Additional CHD risk factors have also been recently identified as unique to women. A history of pregnancy-induced hypertension, gestational diabetes or pre-eclampsia accompanying pregnancy appears to increase the risk for CHD, as do systemic inflammatory illnesses like rheumatoid arthritis and lupus.

Female Hearts Are Different. Women have different heart and artery anatomy and pathology than men. Women's hearts and arteries are smaller. Women more frequently have normal or mildly obstructive coronary arteries than men. When women get angina, they are more likely to have a condition known as microvascular angina. In this case, a coronary angiogram may in fact be completely normal, since the problem lies in the very small blood vessels that penetrate inside the walls of the left ventricle, and not in the major coronary arteries that sit on the surface of the heart.

Women with microvascular angina are often dismissed as not having heart problems, when indeed they suffer from angina pains and may be at risk for heart damage. Such women may needlessly suffer without receiving angina medications or other therapies to reduce their increased CHD risk.

Women are also more likely to develop "broken heart syndrome" than men. This condition is also known as stress cardiomyopathy or by its Japanese name, takotsubo syndrome. It is associated with an extreme emotional or psychological stress (fear, grief, anger, surprise) that triggers a spike in adrenalin and other stress hormones. The sudden release of these hormones is believed to either cause direct damage to the heart muscle or cause profound spasm of the coronary arteries, such that they constrict to a very small caliber. The spasm can cause a marked reduction in the heart's blood supply, which then damages the heart. In either case, the patient can develop chest pain, congestive heart failure and serious arrhythmias. Fortunately, in most cases the damage is temporary and there is a complete recovery.

Female Treatment Differences. The NCEP guidelines for CHD treatment do not differ between men and women. Both genders respond equally to risk management. However, even when women are identified as having CHD risk factors, they are treated with accepted and proven therapies less often compared to men. Women are much less likely to undergo cardiac catheterization, bypass surgery, angioplasty and stent placement than men. Women of equal CHD risk to men are much less likely to receive lipid-lowering treatments and other CHD prevention strategies. The HERS study found that only half of all women with known CHD were on lipid medications.

In the last ten years, while advances in treatment have yielded improved survival rates after a heart attack for men, the death rate in women continues to rise. According to the 2005 Can Rapid Risk Stratification of Unstable Angina Patients Suppress Adverse Outcomes with Early Implementation of the ACC/AHA Guidelines (CRUSADE) registry of 40,000 patients, 35 percent of whom were women, women had a 15 percent higher risk of repeat MI, 30 percent higher risk of stroke and 40 percent higher risk of CHF after an MI than men. These poorer outcomes may have been due to less aggressive treatment in women. Women are 10–20 percent less likely to receive blood thinners, aspirin, ACE inhibitors and statins during and after an MI. Women are 30–40 percent less likely to receive therapies to mechanically open a blocked artery, such as catheterization, angioplasty, stents and bypass surgery. The risk of dying during bypass surgery is twice as high for women as it is for men.

There are a number of reasons for these gender differences. Historically, women have been underrepresented in clinical trials of CHD prevention. Likewise, most trials for CHD treatment have also focused on men. By the last tally, women comprised only 24 percent of participants in all heart-related clinical studies. Another reason is the widely held misconception that CHD risk in women is more time dependent, increasing markedly only after menopause. Finally, since many more women than men present with atypical symptoms, their evaluation and treatment is often delayed, and more aggressive (and potentially heart- and life-saving) therapies are either delayed or underutilized.

Hormone Replacement Therapy. Estrogen is a female hormone that has important physiological functions in women. Receptors for estrogen are located in the breast and reproductive organs, the liver, the cardiovascular system and the bones and skeletal system. Estrogen has several beneficial lipid effects. It increases HDL-C, increases the most protective type of HDL (HDL-2), reduces Lp(a) and reduces LDL-C slightly. However, there are also some negative effects of estrogen on lipids, including a rise in triglyceride levels and CRP. It is no wonder then that the clinical outcomes of estrogen replacement have been mixed and controversial.

For many years the standard of care for all post-menopausal women was to administer hormone replacement therapy (HRT) with synthetic estrogens, such as Premarin, or estrogen and progesterone combinations, like Prempro. Progesterone was added to estrogen to reduce the risk of unopposed estrogen exposure increasing the risk of endometrial cancer. It was believed that replacing diminishing natural estrogen with synthetic estrogen would provide benefits to prevent age-related bone loss, improve cardiovascular well being and treat post-menopausal symptoms like hot flashes, vaginal dryness, mood swings, insomnia and a whole host of other symptoms that occur when estrogen levels decline.

The HERS trial was a secondary prevention trial that studied HRT in nearly 2,000 post-menopausal women with known CHD. It found no benefit to HRT over four years of follow-up. In fact, despite an 11 percent drop in LDL-C and a ten percent rise in HDL-C, HRT caused a 50 percent increase in CHD events during the first year. This difference slowly tapered in later years. Thus, for secondary prevention, HRT was not shown to be beneficial and was actually harmful. The negative effects of HRT extended beyond CHD, as HRT also increased the risk of blood clots and gallstones in the HERS trial's subjects.

The Women's Health Initiative (WHI) study looked at HRT in 17,000 women for primary prevention. While HRT did result in improved blood lipids in women between the ages of 50 and 79 after a five-year follow-up, those receiving HRT had a three percent higher risk of CHD events including MI and stroke. HRT also increased the risk of leg blood clots and breast cancer. There was a modest benefit of HRT in reduced risk of colorectal cancer and bone fractures. Based upon these results, it is now recommended that HRT be given only at the lowest possible dose and for the shortest period of time possible to treat postmenopausal symptoms, but not for primary prevention of CHD.

Closer inspection of these "definitive" trials indicates there were complicating factors that may have skewed the results. Women were not routinely prescribed aspirin for heart, stroke and blood clot protection. The progesterone replacement was one that was later found to counter the protective effects of estrogen. Most women enrolled in the trials were more than 15 years post-menopause and did not have post-menopausal symptoms to warrant the use of HRT.

When the results of the primary prevention WHI trial were analyzed in just those women who were within ten years of menopause, HRT resulted in a 30 percent reduced rate of death, eight percent reduced rate of MI, three percent reduced rate of blood clots and a two percent reduced risk of bone fractures. Even the increased rates of breast cancer and leg blood clots were lower in these women than those women who were started on HRT more than ten years after menopause.

Thus, there may well be a role of HRT in some post-menopausal women. Certainly, if post-menopausal symptoms occur, HRT is indicated to relieve symptoms. In younger women, closer to the onset of menopause, HRT may actually be beneficial. Clearly HRT should be avoided in women who smoke, have a history of blood clots or who have had breast cancer themselves or in their immediate family.

Oral Contraceptives. The currently used low-dose estrogen-progesterone combination oral contraceptives (OC) do not appear to increase or decrease CHD risk. However, if a woman has elevated cholesterol, other significant risk factors (especially smoking) or a current history of CHD, an alternative method to OCs for birth control is suggested, as the risk of blood clots and stroke in such women appears to be increased.

Statins. Although many of the statin trials conducted in the 1990s underrepresented women, subsequent large primary and secondary prevention trials have convincingly demonstrated that women derive the same benefit as men. However, women do pose unique concerns with statins. Women have a higher incidence of muscle aches induced by statins.

During pregnancy, the effects of hormones result in an increase in total cholesterol and LDL-C by 20–25 percent, and a rise in triglycerides by up to 50 percent. However, statins are not to be used in women who are pregnant or might become pregnant, because of the potential risk of harm to the fetus. It is currently recommended that women stop statins for three months before intended pregnancy and remain off medications until they stop breastfeeding. This makes treatment of young women with common genetic lipid disorders such as familial hypercholesterolemia more difficult.

Ethnic Groups

According to the U.S. Census Bureau, by the year 2042 non-Hispanic whites will no longer constitute the majority of the population. Currently, Asian- and Hispanic-origin populations are the fastest growing ethnic segments in every region in the United States. Thus, the need to increase awareness of ethnic issues in CHD is significant. However, even among physicians this awareness is poor. A recent survey of cardiologists found that only one out of three cardiologists acknowledged that there were racial and ethnic cardiovascular-care disparities.

African Americans are two to three times more likely to die of CHD than whites. African American women are 72 percent more likely to have CHD than white women. While blood lipid disorders are less frequent in African Americans, hypertension is more frequently present than in whites or any other ethnic group. African Americans are much less likely to have catheterizations or get stents, clot-buster medications, bypass surgery, cardiac rehab or cholesterol treatment. Overall mortality rates in all forms of heart disease are 10–15 percent higher in African Americans than whites. For African American women, the disparity in treatment and survival rates is even greater.

Hispanics comprise the ethnic segment with the fastest growing rates of CHD in the United States. They are more likely to have triglyceride elevations, diabetes and metabolic syndrome than any other ethnic group. South Asians from the Indian subcontinent (India, Pakistan and Bangladesh) comprise 25 percent of the world's population, yet they contribute to 60 percent of the worldwide burden of CHD. They are second to Hispanics in the incidence of diabetes and metabolic syndrome in the United States. South Asians have levels of Lp(a) that are much higher than they are in the general population, which may in part account for their increased risk of CHD.

Not only are there differences in CHD risk and the level of treatment based upon ethnicity, there are also differences in how various ethnic groups respond to commonly used therapies. For instance, the effectiveness of the anti-clotting medication clopidrogel (Plavix) is strongly affected by ethnicity. Metabolism of this drug is affected by the activity level of the enzyme CYP 2C19. This enzyme in the liver converts clopidrogel into its active form, which can then block platelet clumping and reduce the risk of blood clots. This enzyme functions normally in 98 percent of all whites and in 96 percent of all blacks but is defective in 14 percent of Asians. Tests to determine the activity of CYP 2C19 or the antiplatelet activity of clopidrogel are readily available and should be considered in any patient felt to be at risk for reduced effectiveness of clopidrogel and in all non-Caucasians.

Statins also work differently in various ethnic groups. Blacks typically have a less robust lowering of LDL-C with statin therapy. This is because of altered genetic coding that reduces the effects of stains on the cholesterol-regulating enzyme HMG-CoA reductase. On the other hand, some statins, like rosuvastatin, are metabolized more slowly in Asians. These patients can have very profound effects from statin therapy but may also be more likely to have side effects.

> **Illumination:** At the time of the writing of this book, a large-scale trial called the Multi-Ethnic Study of Atherosclerosis (MESA) is being conducted. Since 2001, this trial has enlisted 7,000 patients of a wide range in ethnicities, without known CHD between the ages of 45 and 85, and is currently following and evaluating these subjects for CHD outcomes. This database is likely to significantly advance our understanding of ethnic differences in CHD.

The Elderly

People over the age of 65 constitute the most rapidly growing segment of our population. Between the increase in prevalence of older individuals, and CHD's predilection to affect older individuals, this segment of our population warrants discussion. For the purposes of lipid management, the NCEP's Adult Treatment Panel Report III (ATP III) defined men 65 and older and women 75 and older as elderly. The estimation of CHD risk in the elderly is no different than that of any other group, except for the fact that by virtue of age itself, these patients all fall into at least an intermediate risk category, meaning their ten-year risk of CHD events is at least ten percent or higher. Risk-reduction clinical trials in both primary and secondary prevention have been conducted and confirm that the benefits observed in patients of all ages was maintained, and in some studies even enhanced, in elderly patients.

A review of 4,000 patients over the age of 65 from the Physician's Health Study who had no known CHD and were followed for nine years found that controlling modifiable risk factors for CHD had a profound effect on the risk of future CHD events. The four modifiable risk factors studied were smoking, non-HDL cholesterol, blood pressure and aspirin use. Control of each risk factor doubled the observed benefit, and when all four risk factors were controlled, the benefit was a four-fold lowering of the risk of CHD events compared to subjects in whom no risk factors were controlled. The Pravastatin in Elderly Individuals at Risk of Vascular Disease (PROSPER) trial looked at 6,000 elderly men and women between the ages of 70 and 82, and found a 15 percent reduced risk of CHD events and a 21 percent reduced risk of death due to heart events after just three years of follow-up in the group of patients who received pravastatin therapy for lipid control compared to a placebo.

One justification for withholding statin therapy in elderly patients has been their shorter life expectancy due to the occurrence of other lethal illnesses like cancer. This is a misconception, as shown by the fact that while 25 percent of patients under the age of 75 die due to CHD, more than 40 percent of patients over the age of 75 die due to CHD. The LIPID study of 9,000 patients aged 65–74 years found statin therapy provided a benefit in older patients that exceeded the benefit seen in younger patients. This was because the shortened life expectancy of older patients was offset by a reduced risk of recurrent CHD events and by shorter durations of hospital stay, both of which tend to be increased in older patients.

> **Alert!** As is the case for women, the risk of muscle side effects with statin therapy is also increased in the elderly. This may be related to a higher incidence of thyroid problems, use of multiple medications or poorer kidney function in older patients. Recently, a higher occurrence of vitamin D deficiency in older patients has also been postulated to be a cause of more muscle problems associated with statin therapy. In such patients, the use of vitamin D supplementation may be beneficial.

Children

Concern about the development of atherosclerosis and subsequent CHD in children continues to increase with the rise in childhood CHD risk factors like obesity, sedentary lifestyles and increasing rates of cigarette use among adolescents. Between the years 1980 and 2007, the incidence of obesity among children has tripled rising, from 10 percent to 30 percent. Obesity is especially prevalent in African American children and teenagers, 10–12 percent of who are classified as being extremely obese. In Mississippi, 44 percent of all children are obese.

Autopsy and pathological studies previously cited in Chapter two, like the Bogalusa Heart Study and PDAY, demonstrate a very high occurrence of atherosclerosis in children and young adults who have died from other causes. Furthermore, the increased recognition of lipid disorders and the genetic susceptibility to CHD in adults has heightened the concerns in these adults that their offspring may also be at risk.

The current NCEP recommendations for the screening of children for lipid disorders are a two-pronged approach: universal and targeted screening. The universal approach focuses on promoting heart-healthy habits and lifestyles for all children beginning at the age of two. These include healthy, low-fat diets of the type promoted by the AHA, physical activity programs and TLC (therapeutic lifestyle changes) measures to reduce CHD risk factors. For children who do not pose additional CHD risk factors, the initial blood lipid screening panel is recommended at the age of 20 years.

In the targeted approach, the same universal TLC recommendations are promoted. However, blood lipid screening is performed in children at the earliest age possible if they are identified as having a family history of early CHD or high cholesterol, or have multiple risk factors such as hypertension, diabetes, obesity, cigarette use, poor diets and/or sedentary lifestyles. Often this approach will uncover many children with previously undiagnosed familial hypercholesterolemia (FH).

Alert! FH occurs in one in 500 children and is more common than sickle-cell anemia and cystic fibrosis. In children at risk for FH, screening blood tests should be done as early as two years of age.

Medication treatment for children with abnormal lipids is only instituted after a trial of TLC interventions, including more aggressive fat-restricted diets and plant sterol and stanol supplements. The target LDL-C in children is under 110 mg/dL. If LDL-C levels remain above 130 mg/dL despite modification of controllable CHD risk factors, medication treatment can be considered as early as ten years of age.

While once considered the first choice of medications for children, the bile acid sequestrants have been replaced by statins as the preferred first-line treatment for lipid abnormalities requiring drug treatment. Statins are much better tolerated and have been studied extensively and found to be both safe and effective in children and adolescents. Both atorvastatin and pravastatin have FDA approval for use in children. In girls of childbearing age, the issue of an increased health risk during pregnancy to the fetus and mother while on statin therapy must be considered.

Other lipid therapies have also been used, but only limited safety and efficacy data are available, and most are not specifically approved for use in children. Ezetemibe is FDA-approved in children over the age of ten as a blocker of absorption of dietary cholesterol and is very well tolerated, albeit a weak agent for LDL-C lowering. Niacin, fibrates and omega-3 fish oil have not been extensively studied and are therefore not approved for use in children.

Acute Coronary Syndrome Patients

Acute coronary syndrome (ACS) refers to the most serious consequence of CHD short of death. Over two million people annually are admitted to coronary care units in the United States with an ACS. In an ACS, a coronary artery blockage, typically due to a combination of atherosclerosis and platelet blood clot, has impaired blood supply to the heart, resulting in either a heart attack or an impending heart attack. Patients with an ACS usually have symptoms such as chest pain, back pain, shortness of breath, nausea or dizziness. They frequently have an ECG that shows signs of reduced blood flow to the heart and also have abnormal blood enzyme levels that signify stress or damage to the left ventricle. ACS encompasses all types of acute heart attacks as well as attacks of severe angina.

Alert! An ACS is a medical emergency that warrants immediate treatment. The mortality rate in ACS in patients who make it to the hospital is six to ten percent. However, up to 50 percent of patients with an ACS will die before they can get to a hospital. Early treatment involves administering aspirin, oxygen, pain killers, blood thinners, nitroglycerin, beta-blockers and often an emergency cardiac catheterization and angioplasty. Opening an occluded artery within 90 minutes (what cardiologists call the "door-to-device" time) of the patient's arrival to the emergency room with an ACS significantly reduces the risk of death and permanent heart injury. Only 15 percent of U.S. hospitals are capable of achieving this standard on a consistent basis.

For the fortunate patient who has survived an ACS, once definitive therapy has been administered to stabilize the patient and restore the blood supply to the heart, the process of secondary prevention begins. This involves a combination of modifying controllable risk factors, taking TLC measures and prescribing medications, as previously discussed. Recent evidence indicates that the primary lipid goal in a patient after an ACS is to reduce the LDL-C quickly and profoundly to 70 mg/dL or less.

The value of high-potency statin therapy early in the course of treatment of ACS is a recent discovery. It was not previously recognized, as early studies on statins excluded patients within the first three to six months of ACS onset. ACS is characterized by a high rate of recurrent cardiac events, particularly within the first six weeks. Up to 20 percent of patients will have recurrent angina, MI, CHF and sudden death, even with therapies such as angioplasty, stents and bypass surgery.

Recent studies using statins early in the course of ACS have found substantial benefit from these treatments. The Myocardial Ischemia Reduction with Acute Cholesterol Lowering (MIRACL) trial used high-dose atorvastatin within 96 hours of ACS and found a 16 percent reduced risk of recurrent CHD events within the first six weeks. These findings were confirmed in both the short-term and long-term in the Pravastatin or Atorvastatin Evaluation and Infection Therapy (PROVE-IT), Aggrastat to Zocor (A to Z) and IDEAL trials.

While patients deriving a benefit in these trials from the use of early high-potency statin therapy experienced a decline in LDL-C levels, the clinical benefits appeared much earlier than could be accounted for by the drop in LDL-C levels. A number of these studies found that CRP levels dropped very early and much more significantly in patients deriving a benefit. This led to the postulate that the early benefits of statin therapy in such patients results from reduced inflammation and the other pleiotropic effects of the statin, like improved endothelial cell function, reduced LDL oxidation and stabilization of vulnerable plaque, and not the lipid-lowering effects. Thus, it is recommended that all patients after an ACS, even those with only mildly elevated LDL-C levels, be placed on high-potency statin therapy.

Alert! Many doctors are not aware that during an ACS the total cholesterol and LDL-C levels are artifactually lower by 10–30 percent than under normal circumstances. Therefore, all patients with an ACS should be placed on statin therapy, regardless of their LDL-C levels.

Chapter 15
Putting It All Together:
Developing and Implementing Your Personalized Program

TIM RUSSERT NEVER regained consciousness after his collapse. Tragically, for his wife of 25 years, the plaque rupture and coronary thrombosis in his left anterior descending coronary artery held true to its nickname, the "widow-maker."

Tim Russert had other significant heart risk factors. His HDL-C had been very low, at 32 mg/dL. His triglycerides were high, at 300 mg/dL. Thus, his non-HDL-C level was elevated, in excess of 120 mg/dL. Russert did not have advanced lipid testing, but the elevated non-HDL-C would indicate he had significantly elevated levels of Apo B100 and LDL particle numbers. It is likely he had a predominance of the atherogenic and dangerous small, dense LDL particles, and not enough of the protective large, buoyant HDL-2 particles. Furthermore, he was prediabetic and overweight, thus likely had the dangerous constellation of atherogenic and metabolic disorders known as metabolic syndrome. It is highly likely he had an elevated level of CRP and evidence of vascular inflammation.

Furthermore, Russert had hypertension, for which he was on medications. He had already developed left ventricular hypertrophy, or a thickened heart muscle, detected on his echocardiogram. He had a coronary artery calcium score of 210 on his cardiac CAT scan, indicating that he already had coronary plaque. He was a high-profile journalist with all of the stress that comes with that job. His Framingham Risk Score predicted he had less than a five percent chance of a CHD event in the next ten years. Clearly his atherogenic lipid profile and other risk factors indicated he was not a low-risk individual.

According to his doctors, Russert was a "model patient" and did everything he was supposed to do. He took his medications, exercised and complied with all of his medical instructions. Treating Tim Russert by the NCEP guidelines did not save his life.

The post-mortem on Tim Russert did not end at the time of his death. Instead, it has become a signature case in the debate about the prevention and management of cardiovascular disease through the accepted and ingrained use of public health policy guidelines versus a personalized and individualized approach. While high-profile cases make the headlines, the reality is that about 300,000 Americans die due to CHD (coronary heart disease) each year in which their first symptom of heart disease was their fatal heart attack. There are an estimated 100,000 Americans who are reassured by their health care providers that they are at "low to moderate risk" even after heart testing and go on each year to have a nonfatal MI, a stroke, an aneurysm or a fatal heart attack.

The NCEP guidelines for the assessment of cardiovascular risk categories, and their subsequent use in treatment plans, are valuable from the standpoint of public health policy. They are formulated by experts who review reams of clinical data from well-designed trials and use evidence-based criteria to develop the guidelines. However, keep in mind that no clinical trial can study patients who have all of the unique medical issues that exist in any given individual. Thus, the guidelines in no way insure that on an individualized basis you will get the best care.

The evaluation and treatment of patients by accepted guidelines is of value for public health policy, in controlling health care costs, and to medical insurers, governmental agencies that supervise and monitor health care quality, physician and hospital "scorecard" makers, and a host of other administrative concerns. However, they are not necessarily the best way for you and your health care provider to approach your unique health care concerns.

Your personal plan to manage your heart risk will involve three things: (1) acquiring the necessary knowledge to understand CHD risk and how it applies to you, (2) understanding the testing procedures to evaluate your CHD risk and, with guidance from your doctor, obtaining those tests that will be useful in assessing your specific risk, and (3) taking the proper steps to lower your future risk of either developing or worsening CHD. The information to develop your personal plan has been presented in this book. It is now up to you to decide how active a role you will take in assimilating this information and then executing the necessary steps in diagnosis and treatment.

Things You Should Know

In order to manage your CHD risk, you need to understand some basic facts and concepts about the healthy heart, cholesterol and heart disease:

☑ The process of atherosclerosis is the same no matter which arteries in the body are affected. In the heart, it is known as coronary heart disease (CHD). In the brain it is known as cerebrovascular disease (CVD). In the legs and aorta it is known as peripheral vascular disease (PVD). In the kidneys it is known as renal artery stenosis (RAS).

☑ The clinical consequences of atherosclerosis result in illnesses unique to the affected artery. For CHD these syndromes are angina, myocardial infarction (MI) and sudden death. For CVD these are stroke (CVA) and transient ischemic attacks (TIA). PVD can lead to claudication, aortic aneurysms, athero-thrombo-embolism and gangrene. RAS can cause hypertension and kidney failure.

☑ Atherosclerosis in all arteries requires four separate but linked processes to occur. These are endothelial dysfunction, cholesterol deposition, arterial inflammation and arterial thrombosis. None of these by themselves are both a necessary and sufficient condition for atherosclerosis to develop. Conversely, prevention and treatment of atherosclerosis needs to be directed toward favorably modifying all of these processes.

☑ Atherosclerosis has significant environmental and genetic influences. In nearly all cases, it is preventable, treatable and even reversible. You must have the proper commitment, knowledge and tools to evaluate and treat your specific condition and risk.

☑ CHD exists in 14,000,000 Americans. Annually, it accounts for over 1,500,000 heart attacks, 500,000 deaths, of which 300,000 occur suddenly and without warning. More people die of CHD than AIDS and all types of cancer combined.

☑ To personalize the statistics, if you are the "average" American:
- You have a one in 20 chance of having significant CHD.
- You have a one in 200 chance of having a heart attack this year.
- You have a one in 500 chance of dying from a heart attack this year.
- In the U.S., a heart attack occurs every 20 seconds, and a death from CHD occurs every minute.

☑ Over half of all patients who suffer an MI never knew that they had CHD. In one out of four patients with an MI, this is their first and last symptom of CHD as they do not survive their MI.

☑ One-half of all victims of sudden cardiac death are under the age of 65.

☑ The likelihood that you have significant CHD can be statistically estimated by knowing your age, sex and whether you are having any symptoms of heart disease. If you have "typical symptoms," this means you have angina occurring when you exert yourself. If you have "no symptoms," this means you never feel chest pain, back pain, arm pain, dizzy spells, fainting episodes, palpitations, and shortness of breath. If you have "atypical symptoms," this means you may have some of these symptoms, but not always with physical exertion.

☑ The following statistical information was published in 1979 in the New England Journal of Medicine from a large database of patients. It indicates the statistical likelihood that significant CHD exists for each designated group:

Age	Typical Symtoms		Atypical Symtoms		No Symptoms	
	M	F	M	F	M	F
40	80%	50%	30%	10%	5%	1%
50	90%	80%	30%	10%	8%	2%
60	95%	90%	50%	35%	8%	2%

See where your age, sex and symptom status put you in terms of your current likelihood of having CHD. Your actual risk may be lower or higher depending on what other risk factors exist. If you have great genetics, and have maintained a heart-healthy lifestyle, your risk will be lower. If you have bad genetics, or have had an unhealthy lifestyle, your risk will be higher. If you are less than 40 or greater than 60 years of age, your risk will be respectively higher or lower than the cut-off ages in this table.

☑ Once you know what your likelihood of having CHD is at this point in time, use a risk-calculator, like the FRS or RRS (see below) to estimate what your risk is of having a cardiovascular event in the next ten years.

☑ The earliest signs of plaque growth, the fatty streak in the coronary arteries, can be found in up to 50 percent of children before the age of 15, and in up to 70 percent of adults before the age of 40.

☑ All types of plaque in the coronary arteries are potentially serious. Most heart attacks occur due to plaque that causes less than 50 percent of the coronary artery to be narrowed. This type of plaque is not detected by most traditional heart examinations and is not treated by heart interventional procedures.

☑ Cholesterol is vital to good health. In the bloodstream, cholesterol is carried by particles called lipoproteins. These are classified according to their density. The main carrier of cholesterol to cells and for its incorporation into arterial plaque is the LDL (low density lipoprotein) particle. The main carrier for removal of cholesterol is the HDL (high density lipoprotein) particle. Thus, LDL-C is known as "bad cholesterol" and HDL-C is known as "good cholesterol."

☑ A variety of important cells, particles and molecules beyond LDL and HDL, play a role in atherosclerosis. These include other lipid particles, inflammatory and thrombotic mediators, as well as white blood cells and platelets.

☑ Plaque in the coronary arteries as well as arteries outside of the heart usually develops and grows silently for years. Plaque growth can ultimately lead to either slow, progressive symptoms or in some cases sudden and catastrophic symptoms. These can include an MI, sudden death, CVA, an aortic dissection or a ruptured aortic aneurysm.

☑ Know your genetics and family history. Any family history of sudden cardiac death or a history of CHD, CVA, PVD or aortic aneurysms in your parents, siblings or children that occurs before the ages of 65 in women and 55 in men is significant.

☑ Although half of all MIs occur in women, women have unique CHD issues:
  • A woman is six times more likely to die of an MI than from breast cancer.
  • A woman under the age of 50 is twice as likely to die of a heart attack as a man of the same age.
  • Adverse changes in blood lipids around the time of menopause significantly increase a woman's risk to develop CHD.

- Sudden cardiac death is 50 percent more common in women having an MI than men.
- Two-thirds of women who die of an MI have no preceding symptoms.
- Women more frequently have "atypical" symptoms during their MI than do men. As a result, women present for medical attention on average, two to four hours later than do men.
- CHD risk factors like obesity, diabetes, metabolic syndrome, HDL-C, triglycerides, CRP and Lp(a) all carry much more importance in women than in men.

☑ African-Americans are twice as likely to die of CHD as whites. African-Americans and women are much less likely to receive life-saving medications and advanced CHD therapies like clot busters, stents and CABG surgery than white men.

Tests You Should Have

Tests to evaluate your heart, circulation and metabolism are necessary to determine the presence and extent of any cardiovascular disease. This testing will determine what level of risk exists within your circulatory system. Do you fall into the category of those needing primary prevention, that is to say there is no evidence that you have any significant CHD or atherosclerosis in any other area? Or, do you fall into the category of those needing secondary prevention, treatment, and reversal? This distinction is crucial in determining the treatment approach that will be necessary for you.

☑ For screening and evaluating your current status and estimating your future CHD risk:
- Fasting lipid panel (total cholesterol, LDL-C, HDL-C, triglycerides).
- Fasting blood sugar.
- Blood and urine tests for kidney function.
- hsCRP level.

- Weight and BMI measurement.
- Blood pressure.
- EKG.
- Chest x-ray.
- Complete medical history and physical examination.

☑ Realistically assess your body fat composition; are you "pear" or "apple" shaped? If "apple" shaped, make weight loss your #1 priority.

☑ Have a risk estimate of the probability that you will have a CHD event in the next ten years using either the Framingham Risk Score (FRS) or the Reynolds Risk Score (RRS). You do not need to do this if you already have CHD, PVD, CVD, AAA, diabetes or kidney disease, since you already fall into a high-risk category, meaning a 20 percent or greater ten-year risk.

☑ Recognize that falling into a "low risk" category does not mean zero risk. Additional tools from blood, genetic and arterial imaging examinations can further refine your individualized risk estimate. Even at low risk, you must still practice preventative strategies for CHD and correct your CHD risk factors.

☑ If you fall into any risk category other than low risk, and you have no symptoms of CHD, discuss testing with your doctor that will look for signs of atherosclerosis in your arteries. The best screening tests for arterial imaging are a carotid ultrasound to measure your cIMT and a cardiac CAT scan to measure your coronary calcium score (CCS).

☑ Advanced lipid testing consists of specialized blood exams that look at more than the traditional lipid measurements in a standard lipid panel. These results can help you refine and personalize your CHD risk estimate. Some of the most important tests in an advanced lipid panel are:
- Apo B100.
- LDL particle number.
- Lp(a).

- LDL and HDL size and density subtypes.
- Lp-PLA$_2$.

☑ Ask your doctor to perform advanced lipid testing if you have any of the following:
- An NCEP risk category of moderate or higher.
- An abnormal cIMT or CCS.
- A family history of premature atherosclerosis.
- Currently on medication treatment for abnormal lipids.

☑ Genetic screening for CHD can test for ApoE, 9p21, and KIF6 genotypes. These tests can provide even more information about your specific risk to develop CHD, as well as what treatments are most likely to be effective to lower your risk. Ask your doctor to perform genetic CHD screening if you have:
- A family history of premature atherosclerosis.
- A moderate to high risk advanced lipid panel.

☑ Have testing for platelet function or your CYP2C19 enzyme status if you take clopidrogel (Plavix) and have had an ACS, CVA or TIA while on this medication. You also need this testing if you are of either African-American or Asian ancestry since you are more likely to be resistant to the anti-clotting effects of Plavix.

☑ Two common causes of premature atherosclerosis and lipid abnormalities in children and young adults are the genetic disorders Familial Hypercholesterolemia (FH) and Familial Combined Hyperlipidemia (FCH). Make sure you are evaluated for both conditions.
- FH occurs in 1/500 persons, and is more common than Cystic Fibrosis or Sickle Cell Anemia. Left untreated, 30–50 percent of individuals with FH will develop CHD before the age of 60.
- FCH occurs in 1/200 persons, and is responsible for 20 percent of the cases of CHD in individuals younger than age 60.

• Both FH and FCH can be transmitted to your children. If you
have either, your children need to be screened at an early age.

☑All children should have a standard lipid panel at the age of 20.
Children with CHD risk factors and/or a strong family history of
premature CHD should have lipid blood tests as early as age two.

☑ Have your vitamin D levels checked if you have either chronic medical
conditions or take statin medications and have minor muscle aches.

☑ Have your testosterone levels checked if you are a man and are experiencing symptoms of "male menopause." If your levels are low, consider
prescription testosterone replacement therapy.

☑ If you have symptoms that are suspicious for CHD, consider more
advanced and sophisticated CHD testing, which can include:
   • Doppler-echocardiography.
   • Stress testing, with or without advanced imaging methods.
   • Multislice cardiac CAT scanning.
   • Cardiac PET or MRI.
   • Cardiac catheterization.

☑ If you are new to a fitness program, consider having a stress test before
you start the program if you:
   • Have significant CHD risk factors.
   • Are over the age of 50.
   • Have any concerning symptoms when you exercise.
   • Have chronic health problems.
   • Take medications to manage CHD risk factors.

☑ If you know you have CHD, undergo screening exams to look for
CVD and PVD.

☑ If you have hypertension, either at an age below 60, or with evidence of kidney abnormalities, or your blood pressures are difficult to control, you should undergo screening for RAS.

☑ If you have CVD, PVD, and/or RAS, undergo advanced testing to look for CHD testing.

☑ If you are a man with ED, or a woman with sexual dysfunction, undergo screening to look for CHD, CVD, PVD and RAS.

☑ Have a thorough dental examination to see if you have gingivitis, putting you at risk for CHD.

☑ If you have joint pains or swelling, be checked to see if you have Rheumatoid Arthritis or other inflammatory disease that increases your risk for CHD.

☑ If you have an abnormal sleep pattern, and especially if you are over-weight, undergo a sleep study to assess for sleep apnea.

Things You Should Do

After you have a good handle on your heart risk and to what extent, if any, your heart has been affected, you can set forth on the path of intervention. Intervention, whether for the purposes of primary prevention, secondary prevention or reversal, will involve steps to reduce your risk of experiencing a heart event, such as an ACS, MI, sudden death, congestive heart failure or arrhythmia. Risk reduction will involve avoiding behaviors that increase your heart risk and embracing actions that reduce your heart risk. Depending on your risk factors and the amount of CHD that may have already developed, medically supervised treatments involving nutrition, supplements, medications, interventions and surgery may be appropriate.

☑ In deciding where to live, pay as much attention to the quality of your health care facilities as you do to the quality of your neighborhood and schools. To make sure you have access to the best cardiovascular care, find out if:

- Your nearest hospital is an accredited stroke center, and can perform 24/7 emergency stroke intervention, that includes emergency thrombolysis (clot-buster medications), interventional radiology and neurosurgery.
- Your nearest hospital is an accredited chest pain with PCI center, and can perform 24/7 emergency catheterization and PCI. If so, make sure the facility has reported its "door-to-device" time (this used to be called "door-to-balloon" time), and that this is consistently less than 90 minutes. If this information is not available publicly, you can locate this from the National Cardiovascular Data Registry (www.ncdr.com).

☑ It matters less which heart-healthy diet you follow, and more whether you actually stick to the diet and "buy-in" to its principles and diet plan. Your target should be to achieve a BMI of less than 26 kg/m². Even modest weight reduction can substantially reduce your CHD risk.

☑ No matter which diet you follow, limit your intake of salt, refined sugar, and starches, cholesterol, trans-fats and saturated fat.

☑ Always select heart-healthy foods. These foods have an abundance of scientific evidence in support of their value:

- Fruits, vegetables and whole grains; pick the ones highest in fiber, have the lowest glycemic-index, and are the closest to their natural state, including unpeeled and unprocessed whenever possible.
- Lean meats, dairy, nuts and legumes for high protein, low saturated fat content.
- Monounsaturated fats, especially olive oil.
- Polyunsaturated fats; especially omega-3 fish or plant oils.

- Alcohol: drink only after approval from your doctor. Men should have no more than 28 grams per day and women 14 grams per day. All types of alcohol have shown a benefit, but red wine, when consumed with meals, appears to be the best.
- Heart-healthy treats, like chocolate, shrimp and green tea.

☑ If your BMI is 27–30 kg/m², consider medical bariatrics and a professionally supervised weight loss program. If your BMI is greater than 35–40 kg/m² and you have failed medical bariatrics, and/or you have a BMI within the range of 30–35 kg/m² and have developed serious health consequences as a result of obesity, consider bariatric surgery.

☑ Exercise regularly, 5–7 days per week for at least 300 minutes per week. Mix in aerobic and light resistance exercises for optimum overall health. You may need to increase the intensity and/or duration of your exercise if weight loss is a priority.

☑ Stop smoking. Get professional help if you cannot do so on your own.

☑ Manage stress in your life.

☑ Maintain a healthy marriage and sexual relationship.

☑ Maintain a healthy sleep pattern of seven to nine hours per day.

☑ If you have acute chest pain, seek medical attention as quickly as possible. Keep the following statistics in mind:
- More than five million Americans visit hospitals each year with chest pain.
- Approximately 70 percent of all cases of chest pain are found to be unrelated to a heart problem.

• Only 50 percent of all patients with an MI will survive before they reach the hospital.
• If you make it to the hospital with your MI, your chance of surviving improves to 94 percent.

☑ If you believe you are having an ACS, chew 160 mg of aspirin and do everything possible to get to an accredited chest pain hospital with 24/7 PCI. Agree to have a PCI if it is recommended.

☑ In most cases, if you have an elective cardiac catheterization (not in the midst of an emergency), you should only agree to have the diagnostic procedure, and not an angioplasty or stent until you have had a chance to get a second opinion.

☑ If your interventional cardiologist recommends a stent, make sure you discuss the following:
• Risks and benefits of a stent compared to medical therapy or CABG surgery in your specific situation. If you are diabetic or have a reduced EF, CABG may be better than stents. Unless you have angina that persists on a good schedule of medications, or are at an imminent risk of having a heart attack, medical therapy is as good as PCI.
• How many stents are anticipated? If multiple stents are needed, CABG might be a better option.
• Will you get a bare metal stent or a drug-eluting stent (DES)? The DES has a lower risk of a recurrent blockage, but requires a more complicated and prolonged blood thinning regimen.
• What antiplatelet medication for blood thinning will you need afterwards and for how long?
• Will an assessment of fractional flow reserve (FFR) be made during the procedure? In a borderline area of blockage, an FFR can eliminate the need for PCI in almost 70 percent of cases.

- Is the interventional cardiologist board certified to perform coronary interventions?
- How many PCI/stent procedures are performed by the cardiologist and the hospital annually, and what are the success and complication rates?

☑ If you are found to have CHD and a CABG procedure is recommended, ask both your cardiologist and the cardiac surgeon the following:

- Risks and benefits of a CABG compared to medical therapy or PCI in your specific situation.
- Is an off-pump CABG or minimally invasive procedure feasible for you? If so, this is a safer and less intrusive option for surgery.
- Is it planned for you to receive a LIMA graft as one of your bypasses? The LIMA lasts longer than vein bypass grafts.
- How many CABG procedures are performed by the surgeon and the hospital annually, and what are the success and complication rates?

☑ If you do not have atherosclerosis in any artery, and have never had a clinical event caused by atherosclerosis, you are a primary prevention patient. You fall into a group of an estimated 100 million other Americans with lipid abnormalities who need primary prevention. Consider the following interventions:

- Therapeutic lifestyle changes to favorably affect diet, weight, exercise and all of your CHD risk factors.
- If you are a woman over the age of 55 or a man over the age of 45, take aspirin at a dose of 81 mg per day, as long as you do not have excessive bleeding or stomach ulcers.
- Take one omega-3 fish oil capsule per day that provides at least 850 mg of combined DHA and EPA content.
- Take a phytosterol supplement at a dose of two to three grams per day.
- Have two to three cups of green tea per day.

- Take vitamin D at a dose of 1000–2000 IU per day if over the age of 50.
- Take immediate release, crystalline niacin supplement at a dose of 500 mg per day if you have a low HDL-C and are not on a statin.
- Consider a red yeast rice supplement up to a dose of 2400 mg per day to treat mild to moderate elevations in LDL-C if you are not on a statin.
- Consider CoQ10 if you take a statin and have minor muscle aches.
- If you are a woman, or have a BMI above 25 kg/m², low HDL-C, diabetes or metabolic syndrome, make sure your triglyceride levels are below 150 mg/dL.
- Consider hormone replacement therapy (HRT) if you are a woman who is less than ten-years post menopause, and have at least a moderately high risk of CHD.

☑ If you already have atherosclerosis in any artery, and/or have had a clinical event caused by atherosclerosis, you are a secondary prevention patient. You fall into a group of an estimated 17 million other Americans. Consider the following interventions, which are in addition to the steps noted above for primary prevention:

- Take a statin to get your LDL-C reduced by 30–50 percent of the values you had when you had your CHD event or from your current levels. At a minimum, the LDL-C levels should be to the recommended NCEP target levels.
- Try and optimize your Apo B100, Lp(a), triglycerides and HDL levels. To do this, you may need other prescription medications in addition to a statin.
- If you have an ACS, make sure you are immediately placed on a statin in the hospital and have a prescription for one upon release, regardless of the results of your lipid blood tests.
- If you have had an MI, CHF or have a reduced EF, make sure you are on a beta blocker.
- If you have had an MI, CHF or have a reduced EF, make sure you are on an ACE inhibitor or ARB.

- If you are a diabetic, make sure you are on an ACE inhibitor.
- If you are a diabetic and have any other CHD factors, make sure you are on a statin.
- Take aspirin at a dose of 160–325 mg per day, unless you take other blood thinners or have bleeding problems or stomach ulcers.
- Consider additional antiplatelet therapy with clopidrogel (Plavix) as it has been shown to reduce the risk of recurrent CHD events as well as improve symptoms in patients with PVD and CVD.
- As a woman, you should not be taking HRT if you have known CHD.

☑ If you are secondary prevention patient, consider the following additional strategies to promote CHD reversal. This is especially applicable to you if you have had a PCI, CABG, MI, CVA, TIA, PVD, RAS or aortic atherosclerosis, since the presence of atherosclerosis in one spot usually signifies that it is developing in other spots as well. Furthermore, after an MI, PCI or CABG, you remain at significantly increased risk for recurrent heart events. Consider the following:

- Within five years of an MI, 18 percent of men and 35 percent of women will suffer another MI.
- Within five years of an MI, four percent of men and six percent of women will experience sudden death.
- Within five years of an MI, 20 percent of patients will develop CHF.
- Consider an Ornish, Pritikin or Portfolio diet to maximize your chance of removing plaque from your arteries.
- Focus on non-dietary measures for cardiovascular health, including aggressive control of your CHD risk factors, a fitness program and stress management.
- Lower your LDL-C to less than 70 mg/dL. Make sure your Apo B100, Lp(a), LDL particle number and LDL density patterns are optimized.
- Raise your HDL-C above 50 mg/dL. Make sure your HDL quality is predominantly the HDL-2 subtype.

A Final Word

Getting the best and most personalized care requires a partnership between you and your health care provider. This starts by selecting a provider who is willing to work on an individualized approach to you and not the "cookbook" approach of blindly following guidelines that the policy makers have introduced into medical care. It continues with you becoming a stakeholder in your medical care. You must become sufficiently well-informed to be an advocate for yourself. You must also buy into making the sometimes difficult choice of changing your lifestyle and having medical testing and treatments that will keep you healthy. If you are willing to make the effort, you will find the reward will be a longer and improved quality of life. Under the guidance of your health care provider, and now armed with the necessary knowledge and motivation, you can take the necessary steps so you **"Don't Let Your Heart Attack!"**

Abbreviations and Acronyms Index

*=Clinical Trial

General Index

ABOUT THE AUTHOR
K. H. Sheikh, MD, MBA, FACC

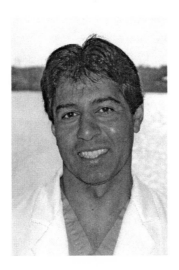

Dr. Sheikh directs a cardiology practice specializing in lipid management and cardiovascular disease prevention and reversal. He practices with Health First Physicians-Cardiovascular Specialists, a single specialty, cardiology practice in Brevard County, on the Space Coast of Florida.

He is board certified in both Internal Medicine and Cardiovascular Diseases. He is a Fellow of the American College of Cardiology. He is a certified clinical lipid specialist, board certified in adult echocardiography and has completed level I training in cardiac CT imaging. His clinical interests include lipid management, comprehensive preventative cardiology, cardiac imaging and invasive cardiology. He was recognized by the Consumers' Research Council of America as one of America's Top Cardiologists.

In addition to his clinical practice, Dr. Sheikh maintains active interests in medical administration, clinical research and teaching. He serves as Director of General Cardiology Services at Cape Canaveral Hospital in Cocoa Beach, Florida. He is a faculty member of the University of Central Florida, College of Medicine. He is also the Director of Clinical Research for Brevard Cardiovascular Research Associates. He is a former Assistant Professor in the College of Medicine of Duke University. He received his MBA from Florida Institute of Technology. He has served as the principal investigator in over 100 national and international clinical trials. He has authored over 150 scientific abstracts, peer-reviewed journal articles, book chapters and subject reviews.

Visit the authors website
http://www.sheikheartcare.com

CPSIA information can be obtained at www.ICGtesting.com
Printed in the USA
LVOW100735181112

307737LV00001B/5/P